Multicultural Issues in Child Care

Second Edition

Janet Gonzalez-Mena
Napa Valley College

Mayfield Publishing Company
Mountain View, California
London • Toronto

Library of Congress Cataloging-in-Publication Data

Gonzalez-Mena, Janet.
    Multicultural issues in child care / Janet Gonzalez-Mena. —2nd ed.
        p.   cm.
    Includes bibliographical references (p.   ) and index.
    ISBN 1-55934-629-9
    1. Child care—United States—Cross-cultural studies. 2. Infants—
Care—United States—Cross-cultural studies.   I. Title.
HQ778.7.U6G663   1996
649'.—dc20   96-20108
                                             CIP

Manufactured in the United States of America
10 9 8 7 6 5 4

Mayfield Publishing Company
1280 Villa Street
Mountain View, California 94041

Sponsoring editor, Franklin C. Graham; production, Publishing Support Services; copyeditor, Michael Ferreira; art director, Jeanne M. Schreiber; cover designer, Joan Greenfield; manufacturing manager, Randy Hurst. The text was set in 10.5/12.5 Janson Text by Publishing Support Services and printed on 50# Butte des Mortes by The Banta Company.

Cover image: © Suzanne Arms

Contents

NOV   1999

Preface

As we approach the twenty-first century, we are forced to make some decisions: Will we honor the diversity present in our early childhood education settings or will we continue to create and implement policies that disregard differences? Will we continue to allow the mismatches between the culture of the family and the culture of the child care center?

Two sample studies—one in California and one in Canada—indicate the need for Canadian and U.S. early childhood educators to respond to diversity. In a California survey of 450 child care centers in five counties, it was found that 96 percent of the surveyed centers serve children from two or more racial groups and 82 percent serve children from two or more language groups.[1] The same survey also found that child care staff are untrained in the cultural matters of the diverse population that they serve.

A similar study in Canada found much the same situation. Information was gathered from 77 child care centers, 199 teachers, 78 schools of Early Childhood Education, and 14 family groups in Montreal, Toronto, and Vancouver. One-third of the teachers interviewed did not believe their training prepared them to work effectively with a diverse population. Many parents and teachers had experienced difficulties in communicating across cultures in early childhood settings.[2]

Further, according to the Toronto *Globe and Mail,*

Ethnic diversity strains day-care staff…Cultural clashes between staff and parents are common as the ethnic diversity of day-care users grows and staff training fails to keep up, says a cross-Canada study. According to Judith Bernhard, author of the study, "right now, (day-care) staff are just guessing at what they should be doing. Their intentions may be good, but the results often are not."[3]

There is a need in Canada and the United States for more training in issues of cultural diversity. Early childhood educators need to broaden their view of appropriate practices to include cultural sensitivity. You'll see that this book is about getting along with people who are different from you, have different ideas about how children grow and develop and how adults and children should behave.

We unconsciously teach the children whose lives we touch about ourselves through everything we do. Though we may seem to be operating out of universal child development principles, the truth is that those principles occur in a cultural context. You can't remove from a cultural framework the ways you relate to children, rear them, determine program curriculum, handle daily routines, and even view the landmarks of physical development. Children learn from their parents, caregivers, and early teachers how to behave in culturally distinct ways. Consciously or not, we work to make the children we care for and teach into the kind of people who fit our culture. It is vital that this process reach the level of awareness. That's what this book is about.

This book serves well as a companion to *Infants, Toddlers, and Caregivers* by Gonzalez-Mena and Eyer (Mayfield, 1996) because of its heavy emphasis on the beginning years. It also fits well as supplementary reading to any child development text because it covers the cultural aspects of development.

This book may also be viewed as a companion to Louise Derman-Sparks's *Antibias Curriculum* (NAEYC, 1989), complementing it nicely. *Multicultural Issues in Child Care* takes off from where Derman-Sparks stopped. Her focus is on an antibias approach to preschool curriculum; the focus here is on an antibias approach to cultural information, adult relations, and conflicts in goals, values, expectations, and child-rearing practices.

This book can be used by anyone involved in teacher training or early childhood education. It serves as a text or supplement for infant-toddler courses; child care and early education classes; supervision and administration classes; social service classes for child care workers; child development and child psychology classes; and Head Start, preschool, child care, and family daycare training.

The material in this book is designed to be practical rather than theoretical; however, theory abounds in the notes following each chapter. The sometimes lengthy notes invite the advanced student to go further and explore themes and issues that are only mentioned in the text.

How This Edition Is Different

This new edition contains more examples of cultural differences and the potential conflicts that can arise. Concrete examples were a feature of the first edition; this edition contains even more. The new references show the burgeoning interest in cultural differences. Native Americans are writing more about their culture and, therefore, they are cited more in this edition than in the last.

An important new feature is the bibliography, which lists many books and articles to help students learn about new ideas and cultures.

Acknowledgments

This edition has been influenced by the knowledge I gained through making a video series on cultural diversity with a multiethnic group. I want to thank the people who helped me complete that project: Magna Systems, Early Childhood Training Series: Diversity, Beverly Aguilar, Dianna Ballesteros, Rose Chou, Susan Dawson, Nancy Ducos, Susan Leong Lee, Lillian Nealy, Intisar Shareef, and Dora Pulido Tobiassen. Special thanks to Shanta and Milan Herzog, coproducers, and to Bill Edwards who made it all possible.

I also want to thank Judith Bernhard, Rich Johnson, Joe Tobin, and Navaz Bhavnagri for stimulating lots of thought about cultural issues and reconceptualizing the early childhood curriculum.

Thanks to BANDTEC (Bay Area Network of Diversity Trainers in Early Childhood) which has broadened my experience with diversity trainers. Thank you to old friends and to some new ones also: Alice Nakahata, Beatriz Leyva-Cutler, Christina Lopez Morgan, Dolores Terrazas, Eleanor Clement Glass, Hedy Chang, Jean Monroe, John Gunnarson, Johnnie McGuire, and Lisa Lee.

I also want to thank Lily Wong Fillmore, Alicia Lieberman, Janice Hale-Benson, Patricia Nourot, Jim Greenman, Anne Stonehouse, and Lyn Fasoli whose writings give me a lot to think about.

I want to acknowledge those at Napa Valley College for their contributions. The staff of the Napa Valley College library was a great help, especially Bonnie Thoreen and Wanda Hass. Thanks to the Napa Valley College child care staff for providing a real life center as a model. Thanks to Maggie Cole, Carolyn Ernst, Kathy Cizek, Debbie Custis, Beverly Aguilar, Elizabeth Karan, Jim Darter, and Socorro Ruiz. Thanks to other Napa Valley College colleagues for more discussion sessions: Carole Kelly Kent, Felicia Shinnamon, Nadine Wade, and Jill Schrutz. Thanks to Tad Parker for continually supporting me.

Special appreciation goes to several people who taught me recently and in the past about cultural differences: Marcus Lopez, Teresa Escobedo, Toni Gomez, Trini Esquivel, Ana Campos, Maria Elena Noriega, Elvira Reyes, Josefina Pacheco, Antonia Lopez, Renata Cooper, Joyce Gerring, Christane Temple, Norma Quan Ong, and Shirley Adams.

I thank those who gave me an antibias perspective: Louise Derman-Sparks, Phyllis Brady, Cecelia Alvarado Kuster, Carol Phillips, and Frances Kendall.

I appreciate the arguments Magda Gerber presented to me to keep me on my toes—also the thinking Sheila Signer, Terry De Martini, Ron Lally, and Peter Mangioni challenged me to do and the warm support of Mary Smithberger.

I also want to acknowledge Enid Elliot, Virginia Dunstan, Joyce Hahn, and Carol Cross for their friendship, support, and feedback.

Thanks to the Mayfield gang, Frank Graham, and Pam Trainer for their support and professional expertise. Also a hearty thanks to my reviewers: Elizabeth Quintero, University of Minnesota-Duluth; Ralph J. Worthing, Delta College, Michigan; and Roberta Bilous, Harrisburg Community College, Pennsylvania. And special thanks to Lynn Graham, Iowa State University of Science and Technology who must have put countless hours into her helpful comments and suggestions.

A big thank you to my grandchildren Shelby and Amanda, and to my children, Tim, Adam, Robin, Bruce, Bret, and Heather who taught me most of what I really know about child development. Most of all, thanks to my husband, Frank Gonzalez-Mena, who made this book possible by taking over more than his share of the parenting and housework for months on end. I appreciate his patience, help, advice, kindness, and willingness to share me with my computer (which he taught me to use). He saw me through this project and I'm grateful.

NOTES

1. Chang, Hedy. *Affirming Children's Roots* (San Francisco: California Tomorrow, 1993).
2. Bernhard, Judith, Lefebvre, Marie Louise, Chud, Gyda, and Lange, Rika. *Paths to Equity: Cultural, Linguistic, and Racial Diversity in Canadian Early Childhood Education* (North York, Ontario: York Lanes Press, 1995).
3. Toronto *Globe and Mail,* January 5, 1996.

To my husband, Frank

What sets worlds in motion is the interplay of differences, their attractions and repulsions. Life is plurality, death is uniformity. By suppressing differences and peculiarities, by eliminating different civilizations and cultures, progress weakens life and favors death. The ideal of a single civilization for everyone, implicit in the cult of progress and technique, impoverishes and mutilates us. Every view of the world that becomes extinct, every culture that disappears, diminishes a possibility of life.

—Octavio Paz

Introduction

This book is about conflict. When cultures collide, we can't just "make nice" and hope the differences will resolve by themselves. We have to first notice them and then we must address them. Many of us trained in early childhood education encounter cultural differences every day and don't even know it. This book is designed to open people's eyes to cultural diversity. After they read this book, many people tell me that they view the world and its people differently than before.

It's wonderful to talk about how we're all different but yet also alike. However, this book isn't about that subject. The reality is that we've got to deal with some tough issues if we're going to respond sensitively to diversity in early childhood programs. The following quote explains why:

> Diversity that somehow constitutes itself as a harmonious ensemble of benign cultural spheres is a conservative and liberal model of multiculturalism that, in my mind, deserves to be jettisoned because, when we try to make culture an undisturbed space of harmony and agreement where social relations exist within cultural forms of uninterrupted accords we subscribe to a form of social amnesia in which we forget that all knowledge is forged in histories that are played out in the field of social antagonisms.[1]

Bell hooks expands on the preceding quote:

> When everyone first began to speak about cultural diversity, it was exciting. Finally, we were all going to break through collective academic denial and acknowledge that the education most of us had received and were giving was not and is never politically neutral.[2]

Hooks explains how painful it was for some in academia to face the loss of their authority as they discovered the limitations of their knowledge. Chaos and confusion arose in the classroom when "universals" were found to be culturally specific. The safe, harmonious, "fun side" of diversity disappeared. Some in academia were distressed. As hooks puts it:

> What they saw happening was not the comforting rainbow coalition where we would all be grouped together in our difference, but everyone wearing the same have-a-nice-day smile.

It's only after we realize that conflict is where growth occurs that we know what we ought to aim for. We need much more training on how to express conflict and then training on how to use effective management and coping strategies to deal with it. We need to know how to restore balance when faced with views different than our own and also to recognize that this balance is always temporary. It is only after we realize that conflict is good and that it won't go away that we will be able to effectively respond to diversity in early childhood teacher training and, therefore, in early childhood classrooms.

As early childhood educators, we need much more training on how to react to a conflict. We need to learn how to put judgment aside and start a dialog based on respect and a willingness to listen.

For example, if a child came to my program with red streaks on her neck and I was told that she was "coined," I'd need to find out more about that procedure before I called the child abuse authorities. If I suspend judgment for awhile, I can make an informed decision about the meaning of the behavior and whether the lasting marks really are injuries. What may be regarded as child abuse by one person may be regarded as a health measure by another.

You may need to trade roles to understand the above situation. Here's an example. What if I moved to a country where they had never heard of immunization? What would be the reaction to sticking needles in a child's arm if no one knew about DPT shots? Would it be fair to accuse me of abusing my children if I gave them shots? At first glance, the practice seems abusive. After all, the preventative nature of the shot can be obscured by the immediate reaction of pain, swelling, fever, and general malaise. I believe I am protecting my children when I get them immunized, even if the effect is negative for a few days. It is important to take your time in judging parents who rub coins on their children's necks for health reasons. You may not understand the purpose of the practice.

Of course, one must not abandon judgment permanently. For example, if I were a caregiver in a dialog with a parent who was telling me to put her baby to sleep in a prone position, I couldn't just listen and agree. I couldn't reassure myself that it's best to put babies to sleep in the way they are used to. It is my responsibility to mention to this family the research on Sudden Infant Death Syndrome (SIDS). A prone sleeping position isn't safe. The same applies to putting a baby to bed with a bottle. Parents need to be made aware of the possible consequences of such practices.

The difficult aspect of a conflict situation in a child care setting is that most practices don't have obvious consequences or proven risks. In other words, they aren't clearly right or clearly wrong. Differences in practices often depend on differences in priorities. There are times when we get ourselves in situations where we believe so strongly that we are right that we can't see the other person's view. We, of course, can only see the world through our own eyes. It takes imagination to see another person's view. Most of us need help in increasing our imagination. This book is designed to give you that help.

This book is also designed to express the message that in a conflict situation—when two views oppose each other—it doesn't mean one is wrong and one is right. As early childhood educators we should all practice saying on a regular basis, "I'm not saying you're wrong; I'm just saying I disagree with you."

One basic area of difference is the conflict between independence and interdependence goals. Independence and individuality are considered universal goals in most early childhood training programs. As a European-American, I believe in promoting independence and individuality. My understanding of child development leads me to promote independence and individuality. However, I am aware that other cultures downplay independence and individuality. If I have families in my program whose priorities are different from mine, I must respect the differences. I must also work with those families to figure out WHAT TO DO about our differences. What practices reflect independence goals? What practices reflect interdependence goals? What practices promote individuality? What practices promote embeddedness in the group? These are important questions to answer if you are a teacher working in a cross-cultural situation. This book is designed to help you start asking these questions.

Getting answers to those questions involves interacting in real-life settings. The problem is that many early childhood educators are more likely to either ignore problem situations or to argue about them. The kind of interaction needed is called *dialog*. Dialoging is different from arguing. Arguing has persuasion behind it. We argue to win somebody over to our side. However, in dialoging, rather than trying to convince someone of their own viewpoint, people try to understand the other perspective. The idea is not to win, but to find the best solution for all people involved in the conflict.

Here's a summary of the differences between an argument and a dialog:

- The object of an argument is to win; the object of a dialog is to gather information.
- The arguer tells; the dialoger asks.
- The arguer tries to persuade; the dialoger tries to learn.
- The arguer tries to convince; the dialoger tries to discover.

- The arguer sees two opposing views and considers hers the valid or best one; the dialoger is willing to understand multiple viewpoints.

When faced with a conflict or problem, the natural reaction of most people isn't to start a dialog. Speaking for myself, once I begin to address a problem or conflict, I'm likely to start arguing. When I do that, I'm always so anxious to win that I begin to make assumptions and to jump too quickly to conclusions. When I argue, I try imposing my own solutions without listening carefully to the other person. Sometimes, the other solutions are as good or even better than mine. I could save a lot of emotional energy and, perhaps, damaged relationships if I avoided the argument and focused on trying to create a dialog.

During several videotape sessions in which a group of early childhood educators role played parents and teachers in conflict, I saw that others tend to argue the same way that I do. After watching those tapes repeatedly, I began to notice that people used certain types of body language when they tried to express the correctness of their views to the other person. They tended to stand firm and tough, with a defensive position, when listening to the other person. When it was their turn to talk, they leaned forward and made cutting or pushing gestures with their hands. Just by looking at each person, you could tell that they were fighting about something. Without even listening to what they were saying, it was obvious that they were in a potential win-lose situation.

Dialoging is very different from arguing. I also got to see examples of dialoging in those role plays and the difference was evident in body language. I saw people who were also equally emotional and firm in their stances; however, they used their bodies and voices differently. Their purpose was to hear the voice of the other person. Their gestures reflected their attitude, hands especially. Instead of waving fists or making strong pushing or cutting movements, their hands tended to be open. The open hands was a reflection of the open mind— or maybe it was the reverse.

So, how does one switch from an argument to a dialog in the heat of the moment? Start by noticing your body language. Sometimes by just changing your body language you can switch your energy. After that, it's a simple thing: listen to the other person. To truly listen, one must suspend judgments and, instead, focus on what's being said. Really hearing someone is extremely simple, but it's not easy.

"I don't need the kind of training you're talking about," some early childhood educators tell me. "I don't have diversity in my program. The families I work with all come from the same ethnic background." My answer is: every program has diversity. Sometimes it shows, sometimes it doesn't. I've seen and experienced many arguments among staff or between staff and parents even when there was no obvious cultural diversity. One example (and I could give hundreds) was an argument between a family and a program that were racially and ethnically similar. The family followed a strict vegetarian diet, which caused many problems for the teachers who didn't know what the family wanted for their child. The misunderstandings would have been easier to accept if the parent had come from another country, had dressed in exotic clothes, and had a religious reason for their preferences. Although clear cultural differences are present in some child care settings, less obvious individual differences are always present, even in settings where everyone seems to come from the same background.

The supreme challenge of this book is to give specifics of both clear and not so clear cultural differences without giving misinformation. The issue that confronted me as I worked on this book is truth. How could I tell the truth about culture when it is such a slippery subject? I addressed this challenge by using several approaches.

I used my own personal experience whenever possible. My experience isn't valid for everybody, but it's true for me. I also used *stories*—some of which were true and some of which were based on truth but stretched to fit the situation. Story telling provides a basis for the reader to create truth as well as to understand a point in a different way from academic discourse.

Most importantly, I used information and quotes from direct sources as much as possible. I let people talk about their own culture. You'll see in the bibliography that I searched for books and articles by writers who belong to the culture they write about. Some are less academic than others. Some of the book publishers are small and less known than others.

Remember, knowing something about a culture doesn't mean that you can predict how a person from that culture will behave in a given situation. We must be very careful about generalizations. There are enough stereotypes in the world now—let's not add to them.

When I began writing this book, I used all of my experiences in cross-cultural exchanges and my readings in anthropology, linguistics, and communication theory, particularly intercultural communication. I had to look outside my own discipline of child development to get a broader picture of cultural diversity.

But, even with all the studying, I didn't understand the full picture until I discovered the antibias curriculum developed by Louise Derman-Sparks and her Antibias Curriculum Task Force. *The Antibias Curriculum* does not pertain to infants, which is a subject of major interest to me, and there's only one chapter on adult relations, but the spirit of Derman-Sparks' book inspired me to look for my own meanings of antibias curriculum.

The particular message I took from her book and expanded in my book is this: If you continue to follow your own ideas about what's good and right for children in child care, even if those ideas are a result of your training, you may be doing a disservice to children whose parents may disagree with you.

This book is about conflict. That's what makes it so interesting. This book asks more questions than it answers. That's what makes it frustrating. Reading this book is not a neutral experience.

NOTES

1. McLaren, Peter. "Critical Multiculturalism and Democratic Schooling" in the *International Journal of Educational Reform*, quoted in bell hooks, *Teaching to Transgress*. N. Y.: Routledge, 1994.
2. Hooks, bell. *Teaching to Transgress*. N. Y.: Routledge, 1994.

CHAPTER ONE

Perceiving and Responding to Differences

A s a white, middle-class American with mostly Anglo-Saxon heritage (my Spanish surname comes from my husband), I was surprised to discover that I have a culture. I have learned that I unknowingly move within a cultural framework every minute of every day. That framework influences the way I think and act and how I perceive, handle, and interact with people and materials. It determines my notions of time and space and even influences my behaviors related to those notions.[1]

CULTURE IS UNCONSCIOUS

I move within this cultural framework as unconsciously as I move within the physical world I live in. I don't think about putting one foot in front of another when I walk. I don't think about my culturally determined actions, postures, ways of dealing with people—they're automatic.

When I meet someone who obviously doesn't move in the same cultural framework that I do, I'm jarred. Because my way seems right, even normal, I tend to judge others based on my own perspective. I may consider them exotic or interesting, or I may consider them weird. But being a polite person who tries to get along with people, I do what I can not to notice. Because my way is normal to me, it seems rude to make an issue of the fact that someone else is not normal. And because I have a whole society behind me giving me the message that "my people" are the standard by which everyone else is judged, I can afford to keep on ignoring what I chose to.

A Narrow View

But can I? What does this attitude do to me? It shields me from reality. It gives me a slanted perspective, a narrow view. I miss out on a lot because of my perspective. Besides, it gives me a false impression of importance, letting me believe that "my people" are the only ones who count in the world, where in reality white, middle-class, Anglo-Americans like me are a small minority of the world population.

What does it do to those who are not "my people" if I continue in this narrow, slanted perspective, ignoring what I consider "not normal"? I train teachers and educate parents; therefore, I have a lot of influence over the next generation. Imagine the harm I can do both to "my people" and those whose differences I ignore when I carry out my job with this biased attitude. Imagine what my students can do to the children they live and work with when they define "normality" in the narrow ways they learn from me. What does it do to people who are different from me to have those differences defined as abnormal? What does it do to people who are different from me to have those differences ignored?

What Are the Effects of Being Ignored?

That's an important question: What does it do to someone to ignore some integral aspect of his or her identity?

My husband was born and raised in Mexico. Every now and then someone says to him, "I never think of you as being Mexican." They mean this as a compliment. Because I'm not Mexican, I don't know how this feels. But I can imagine how I would feel if someone complimented me by saying he never thinks of me as a woman. That would shock me because being female is a vital part of who I am, and I don't want to be considered genderless. I don't want anyone to stereotype me because I'm female. I don't want anyone to hold my gender against me or treat me unequally either, but I would feel very strange if someone made a point of ignoring a vital part of my identity.

Broadening Our View

This book is an attempt on my part to broaden my own perspective of what's normal—to quit applying a single standard for adaptive, healthy, and competent behaviors. I have a strong desire to quit ignoring differences and begin not only to notice them but to celebrate them. I want to look at differences as sources of strength, not abnormalities or weaknesses. I don't expect to change all at once—in fact, I've been working on this shift of perspective for a number of years. Revising one's views can be a slow process.

CULTURAL PLURALISM

In less personal terms, the ideology on which this book is based is *cultural pluralism*. Cultural pluralism is the notion that groups should be allowed, even encouraged, to hold on to what gives them their unique identities while maintaining their membership in the larger social framework. Mutual respect is the goal, though it isn't easy because, at least in the human development/education fields, we've been taught a deficit model where intellectual, family, and mental health practices that differ from the mainstream, middle-class norm are not viewed as cultural differences but as defects or inadequacies. Similarly viewed were behaviors that are competent and adaptive responses to a history of bias and misunderstanding in a society that has always had first and second class citizens. We have all been subjected to a good number of misunderstandings in the past. This book is an attempt to correct some of them.

Cultural Pluralism and Child Care

You can't remove from your cultural framework the ways you relate to children and manage their behavior, plan a curriculum, set up the environment, handle caregiving routines, and carry out parent education. Your behaviors are determined by your values, which are cultural, familial, and individual.

To aim for cultural pluralism in a child care program, one must have a clear understanding of differences. One must see where child and teacher behavior fail to mesh so that adjustments can be made. One must know and respond to the parents' goals, values, and beliefs related to the care of their children. One must know how to meet the needs in culturally appropriate ways.

It may seem that cultural differences have little to do with the nitty gritty of meeting children's needs. After all, how many different ways can there be to feed, clean, carry, dress, and touch children and provide for rest and warmth? Where do the cultural differences come in?

The differences show up in *the way* the needs are met—in how teachers and caregivers interact and relate to children, in the issue of body language and non-verbal communication. Culture is learned very early, and early childhood theoreticians and practitioners can't afford to ignore this fact.

Babies Are Raised to be Members of Their Culture

Look at an example of a difference in the way that two cultures relate to their babies. The difference reflects what the adults in each culture believe is good for babies, which in turn reflects their varying value systems. Here's the example. When comparing three to four month old infants in middle-class homes in Japan and America, Caudill found American mothers (he means white, European-

American mothers) talked to their babies more, and Japanese mothers spent a good deal of time lulling and soothing their babies. The Americans were stimulating their babies. The Japanese were doing the opposite.[2]

So what? What does it matter if some parents spend more time stimulating their babies and others spend more time calming them? It matters a lot because how the adults treat babies affects those babies' behavior and personality development.

As Caudill found, the result of the differential treatment was that the American babies were more physically and vocally active, and the Japanese babies were less so. Caudill concluded, *"Thus, because of the different styles of caretaking in the two cultures, it appears that by three to four months of age infants have already learned (or have been conditioned) to behave in culturally distinctive ways and that this has happened outside awareness and well before the development of language"* (emphasis added).[3] In other words, the European-American mothers were making their babies into the kind of people who would fit their culture, and the Japanese mothers were doing the same.

Think about what might happen if the babies were handled some of the time by European-American mothers and some of the time by Japanese mothers. They might come out to be bicultural people, compartmentalizing their differential treatment. Children do that—they know they are treated one way by this person in this setting and another way by another person in another setting. However, instead of becoming bicultural, they might instead become confused about how they are supposed to be. If this is the case, the environment with the "foreign mother" might be called culturally assaultive. ✓

Babies and young children become acculturated to the distinct individual and cultural rhythms of their teachers and caregivers. They learn synchrony that in some cases seems to be culturally specific.

Synchrony Is Important

An interesting analysis done by Byers and Byers of a videotape of a small group of nursery school children showed an African-American child who consistently failed to get her teacher's attention because she was out of synch with the white teacher's "scanning behavior."[4] Although it seems like a small thing, failing to get a teacher's attention can eventually impact on how a child feels about herself. She may wonder why she never gets to talk in a group situation or answer the teacher's questions. Does the teacher dislike her? Is the teacher discounting her? Is she not as smart as the other children? Let's assume that the problem was simply a mismatch between the teacher's scanning behavior and the child's attention-getting behavior. It would be important for the teacher to learn to get more in synch with this child. It would also be important to empower the child in the teacher's culture. Cultural learning is a two-way street. However, it's important that a child not lose her own culture while becoming empowered in the mainstream culture. Cultural identity and family connectedness are vital for emotional health.

You may be thinking that the teacher is ignoring the child on purpose. There's no denying that racism can be a factor in teacher–child interactions. It's always possible that conscious or unconscious bias play a role in the teacher's "scanning behavior." Sometimes a teacher's behavior is a matter of lack of understanding or skills; other times deeply held attitudes are the problem.

Attitudes are harder to change than lack of skills. However, knowledge and awareness can help. That's where training comes in.

Misunderstandings

For years I have been teaching about three parenting styles called (among other things) permissive, authoritarian, and authoritative. The research behind this way of looking at parenting made perfect sense to me.[5] I have seen the problems that occur when children have authoritarian parents. I know that controlling and restrictive child-rearing practices predict poor school achievement. What I didn't see was the fact that I was looking at European-American children. Then I read an article by Ruth Chao describing a "paradox" involving the child-rearing practices of Asian parents. Chinese parents are authoritarian, but their children don't exhibit poor school achievement! In fact, they do very well in school. Chao's article broadened my view appreciably. I never considered before that the concept of authoritarianism may have very different meaning depending on the culture. I also never thought about the historical context of authority in this country. As a nation that started with a rebellion against authority, we have a legacy of ambivalence surrounding the concept. The idea of and feelings about authority in other countries is different. When Chinese children are being "controlled" and "restricted," they see their parents' behavior differently from the way European-American children see their parents' controlling behavior.

Understanding cultural differences is a subject that goes far beyond what holidays people celebrate and what foods they eat.

More Examples of Cultural Differences

Jim Greenman provides an example of a program designed to be culturally sensitive that ran into a problem.

"There has been an influx of Hmong people from Laos and Cambodia to Minnesota. A child care center with many Hmong children was trying to improve the infant and toddler program by hiring more Hmong staff. The center believed in a language-rich environment and much personal one-to-one interaction between caregiver and baby. With Hmong staff, they got very little language and very little interaction." This situation provides a very real example of a conflict of style in relating to babies. Greenman goes on to explain. He starts by examining the customs that result in the differences in style. "What would be normal in Hmong society? Mothers strap their babies to them, and this happened at the center. They have constant bodily interaction but not the interaction we know."[6]

But this book isn't just about foreigners who come to this country and discover cultural conflicts. It's also about Canadians and Americans who find themselves in conflict with other Canadians and Americans over cultural differences. These conflicts are in some ways even harder to deal with because of an attitude that says "when in Canada and America, do as the Canadians and Americans do," which, of course, is a meaningless statement unless you define *which* Canadians and Americans you're talking about. It's also harder to deal with because so many believe that "American" means white, European-American, and middle class— taking the "white-is-right" attitude. A further problem is that differences among Americans aren't always defined as *cultural* differences.

Greenman gives a further example, which relates to experiences I have also had in child care. He tells the story of some African-American parents who complained about sand in their children's hair:

> I worked in a center that believed kids should get dirty and be little scientists—it had a wonderful adventure playground. Parents, particularly black parents, would say: "We don't want our kids going outside. We spend an hour and a half on their hair. Two minutes later they are covered with sand. We can't get that stuff out and we spend our whole evening cleaning it up. So we don't want our kids going outside." For awhile, our earnest and empathic response was: "Gee, that's too bad. But this really is good for the children." Of course our knowing response implied, "You poor, ignorant person, valuing appearance over good child development." Conflict continued and we learned. Now the response to these sorts of issues is: "Okay, let's figure this out. Obviously it's important to you how your child looks. And you know it's very good for children to have these sorts of experiences. Let's come up with a solution." The assumption is two legitimate points of view—let's work it out together. In this instance, the answer was shower caps for the kids.[7]

"Let's Figure This Out"

So if you're not going to just say, "This is how we do it here in our program, and you'd better learn our ways," what do you do? You start by treating the different perspectives as equally valid. When you come from that point of view, you can do some problem solving around the issue and together come up with a solution—like the shower cap one. There's more about that in Chapter Two.

One reason I wrote this book was to help me and others become aware of and sort out these conflicts. I need help to listen. I know others do too. A quote from Lisa D. Delpit brings this point home. She quotes an African-American who is lamenting what happens in discussions about what is best for African-American children: "When you're talking to White people they still want it to be their way.

You can try to talk to them and give them examples, but they're headstrong, they think they know what's best for *everybody*, for *everybody's* children. They won't listen, White folks are going to do what they want to do anyway."[8] I think back on the times when I've been one of those "White women who wouldn't listen," or maybe I listened, but I couldn't hear.

The goal is for adults to discuss potential conflicts and learn to dialog about them so that children in child care experience fewer harmful conflicts in approach when the teacher or caregiver and parents disagree about what's good or right. It's important for teachers or caregivers to clarify what they believe is good practice, as well as begin to open up to other perspectives—even those that may conflict with their own.

A CONTRAST IN VALUES

It's extremely difficult to understand the perspective of someone else—especially when it conflicts with your own. One of the reasons why I can't hear or understand someone who is different from me is that I have no perception of the value system. For example, if a mother insists on spoon-feeding a child who is quite capable of feeding herself, I feel upset. Until I understand that she values dependence, we'll have a hard time talking to each other!

How someone can value dependence was a question I asked myself when I first heard of such a thing. To me, being dependent is something to be avoided whenever possible. Of course, I am dependent in many areas of my life, but I don't feel good about it.

It has been hard for me to understand that dependence is something desired and even sought after by some cultures. In fact, some families *train* their children in dependence as well as independence. Joe Tobin, coauthor of *Preschool in Three Cultures*, told me about lessons in dependence he discovered in Japan. These lessons begin about the time babies start trying to do things for themselves. The idea is to teach children to "graciously receive help." A friend of mine from Taiwan, Rose Chou, explained the concept again to me. Whenever she visits her grandmother, Rose lets her grandmother care for her and do things for her because it makes her grandmother happy.

According to Edward Stewart, cultures other than Asian see dependence differently from the way American and Canadian mainstream cultures do: "Dependence is not deplored by the Latin as it is by Americans."

He also explains why dependence is valued: "Dependence on others is desirable, for it strengthens the relationship among people." Stewart broadens the example Rose Chou gave me by reversing it: "Chinese parents take pride in being dependent on their children and supported by them in a manner to which they are unaccustomed.[9]

By giving cultural information such as this, and by putting cultural labels on people and behavior, I run the risk of promoting stereotypes that already exist and perhaps even creating some new ones. Upon looking at the literature, I've discovered biased ways of reporting results of research that compare cultures in negative ways. It's easy for me to do that too, without even realizing it. When I lift facts out of their context or behaviors out of their cultures or environments, I'm in danger of confusing the issues. And if I speculate where certain practices came from, I'm in danger of being wrong. After all, very few parents can explain why they do what they do with their children, if they even recognize they are doing it at all. Many child care practices are handed down generation after generation and aren't explained in terms of adaptation for survival of the species and the culture.

Cultural labels are necessarily generalizations. As soon as I mention a reference that talks about the Chinese, for example, a good number of people who identify themselves as Chinese will say, "I'm not like that" or "I don't have that value." If "Mexicans" are compared to "Americans," that's a gross generalization. Which "Mexicans"? Which "Americans"? You have to consider age, income level, geographical location, ethnicity, family origins, history, dynamics, and a whole lot more. Then even after you find two families who are the same in all these factors, individuals in that family may differ drastically from each other. My sister and I are nearly the same age, from the same culture, and were raised in the same family; yet we don't agree about what's good for children.

Even when one is being supersensitive to all the problems in understanding cultural differences I've mentioned, the job is still hard because cultures are constantly changing—especially as they come in contact with other cultures. It's important to recognize that the culture of a first-generation Vietnamese or Hmong immigrant, for example, is different from a second- or third-generation member. The culture changes when it comes to this country, even in families trying hard to preserve it. Someone who is Puerto Rican from New York is different from a Puerto Rican from Puerto Rico.

So what can one do when faced with all this confusion about labels and culture? Don't throw out cultural differences as a valid concept, but look at people as people. No matter what culture a person comes from, a goal should be to develop a person-to-person relationship. Treating people with respect solves many cross-cultural problems.

I've tried to minimize the mistakes by dealing whenever possible with conflicts in themes and trends. My original intention was to describe only conflicts, not cultures, so I tried to contrast cultures without naming them. I didn't want to categorize and label. I was trying to avoid a tendency of my culture: to analyze everything and put it into boxes. My goal was to raise questions rather than provide answers. But I got so much pressure to be more specific as I used the various drafts of this book in my classes and workshops that I gave in and decided to provide references and examples. By doing that, I know I will offend those who find their culture pictured in what seems to them an unflattering way. I know sensitive people will find bias in what I've chosen to include and eliminate. I know some won't relate to what I say here about their culture. I'm sorry. I know I will step on toes, but my hope is that more good will come out of it than harm.

This chapter has looked at cultural differences in order to promote a particular message. Adults working with children and parents in child care settings need to regard sensitivity, respect, communication, and problem solving as keys to providing what children need. I propose we each work hard to reconcile differences in beliefs while tuning in to the individual needs of each child in our care in ways that promote his or her own culture.

What's Good for Children: A Multiethnic View

It's good for children to receive **culturally competent care** that is **sensitive** and has a **global, multiethnic view.**

Culturally competent care **requires** that:

- Adults in children's lives respect each other.
- Adults in children's lives work to understand each other's perspectives.
- Caregivers and parents understand how program and family values may differ and work together toward blending differing value systems.
- Adults in children's lives create **ongoing dialogues.**

Dialogues

- Dialogues ensure that information exchange occurs so that good judgment can result from the blending of shared points of view.
- Dialogues mean that everyone who works with children is both a teacher and a learner. Caregivers must be willing to understand each other and to view parents as the experts who know what's good for their children.
- Dialogues occur when the people in question begin by listening to each other instead of judging.

Transformative Education

- **From respectful interactions and ongoing dialogues comes transformative education.** When we acknowledge that our experiences with one another are important, when we stretch to understand different points of view, we become transformed by each other's life experiences to a different level of knowledge and sensitive multiethnic care. **That's good for** children!

If we are continually open and sensitive, we will encounter dilemmas. Most of the time there is no one answer, only a continual process of dialog. My newest dilemma concerns babies and sleeping positions. If one is to be both culturally sensitive and wise, one must confront the fact that new research shows that SIDS (Sudden Infant Death Syndrome or "crib death") risk increases when babies are put to sleep on their stomachs.[10] Yet how many parents, for individual and cultural reasons, prefer that their babies sleep in a prone position? You have to talk about it!

FOR FURTHER READING

Hall, Edward T., *Beyond Culture*. Garden City, N. Y.: Anchor Books, 1977. An eye-opening book about hidden culture and differences.

Carroll, Raymonde, *Cultural Misunderstandings: The French-American Experience*. Chicago: University of Chicago Press, 1988. Not specifically about early childhood, but helps mainstream middle-class North American readers perceive their own culture when it contrasts to another.

Clark, A. L., ed. *Culture and Childrearing*. Philadelphia: F. A. Davis, 1981. Gives a good overview of child-rearing practices as described by members of various cultures.

Gonzalez-Mena, Janet, "Do You Have Cultural Tunnel Vision?" *Child Care Information Exchange*, July/August 1991, pp. 29–31. About perceiving differences and is aimed specifically at a child care audience.

Greenman, Jim, "Living in the Real World: Diversity and Conflict." *Exchange*, October 1989. Jim Greenman provides examples from child care settings that help make it easier to perceive and know how to respond to differences.

NOTES

1. Hall, Edward T., *Beyond Culture*. Garden City, N.Y.: Anchor Books, 1977, p. 42.
2. Caudill, William, and Frost, Lois, "A Comparison of Maternal Care and Infant Behavior in Japanese-American, American, and Japanese Families," *Youth, Socialization, and Mental Health*, vol. 3 of *Mental Health Research in Asia and the Pacific*, William P. Lebra, ed. Honolulu: University Press of Hawaii, 1974, p. 3.
3. Ibid.
4. Byers, P. and Byers, H., 1974, reported in Lubeck, Sally, *The Sandbox Society: Early Education in Black and White America*. Philadelphia: Falmer Press, 1985, p. 36.
5. Baumrind, Diana, "Current Patterns of Parental Authority," *Developmental Psychology*, 4(1), 1971, pp. 1–103.
6. Greenman, Jim, "Living in the Real World: Diversity and Conflict," *Exchange*, October 1989, p. 11.

7. Ibid., p. 13.

8. Delpit, Lisa D., *Harvard Educational Review* 58(3), August 1988, 280–297.

9. Stewart, Edward C., *American Cultural Patterns: A Cross-Cultural Perspective.* Yarmouth, Maine: Intercultural Press, 1972, 72.

10. Beal, S. M. and Finch, C.F., "An Overview of Retrospective Case Control Slides Investigating the Relationship Between Prone Sleeping Positions and SIDS," *Journal of Pediatrics and Child Health* 27, 1993, pp. 334–339.

CHAPTER TWO

Communicating Across Cultures

I once sat by a window looking out across the street at a man who was acting very strange. I could see him only from the waist up, but that was enough for me to know he was making extraordinary gestures and facial expressions. I opened the window so I could hear his words. I was even more mystified. The words coming out of his mouth were in a language I didn't understand, and they sounded very strange indeed. I watched this man for sometime, trying to figure out what he was doing walking back and forth on the sidewalk making weird gestures and sounds. I had decided he was crazy and had begun to feel afraid when finally I stood up and saw the whole picture. There at the man's heels was a dog. Immediately everything made sense. Aha, he's training a dog, I said to myself. I would have figured it out sooner if this man had been of my culture and used the command facial expressions, gestures, and, especially, the words I was familiar with. I learned two lessons from this experience: (1) You may have to see the whole picture to understand. (2) It's important to know the meanings attached to the behavior.

INTERPRETING THE MEANING OF BEHAVIOR

This man training dog incident was a simple cross-cultural experience. It wasn't even an encounter—I was a mere observer. Once I saw the whole picture, I could deduce the meaning of the behavior. In most cross-cultural encounters, it isn't that simple. The meaning you attach to the behavior may not be even remotely related to the meaning the person you're encountering puts on it. A smile may not mean friendliness or even happiness; it may mean embarrassment. When you combine words, gestures, facial expressions, timing, proximity, and all the other parts of an exchange, the meanings become even more complex.

In any cross-cultural exchange, it is vital that you find out what meanings the behaviors have to the person performing them rather than doing what is natural—assigning meanings and values to the behavior of others based on your own culture. It is also vital to understand that your behavior doesn't necessarily convey your own meanings and values to the other person.

THE IMPORTANCE OF TEACHERS' AND CAREGIVERS' UNDERSTANDING CROSS-CULTURAL COMMUNICATION

In this wonderfully diverse continent of ours, teachers and caregivers encounter cross-cultural exchanges every day as they care for children whose cultures are different from their own. I don't mean just immigrant children from, say, Southeast Asia, but also children of past immigrants who have been arriving in this country for the last two hundred fifty years from all over the world. I'm also talking about the original Canadians and Americans who were here first. Though all are Canadians and Americans, we don't share a single culture. Our rich variety of cultures in Canada and America makes us who we are. It also complicates and enriches the job of teachers and caregivers as they strive to learn to communicate, understand, and respect the values and child care practices of parents of cultures different from their own.

Child care is a rapidly growing institution, and infant care is the fastest growing aspect of it. The children being cared for are increasingly of ethnic minority groups as the Canadian and American populations move toward the majority becoming a minority.

The fact that more and more infants are being cared for outside their own homes is significant considering the trend of increasing cultural diversity. Infants are still developing their identity. They have little sense of self or cultural identity and few cultural skills. They develop their identity and learn their cultural skills from those around them. They are different from the four or five year olds who arrive in child care already knowing who they are, what culture they belong to, and who have cultural skills. Their developing sense of identity is already beginning to form. The main concern for preschoolers is to keep from harming their self-esteem and cultural connections.

It's important for all children to have strong positive models from their own culture. It's especially important for infants.[1]

Child-rearing practices and the beliefs, goals, and values behind them are deeply tied to culture. As long as parents can find people to care for their children who agree with them about child-rearing practice, there's no problem. Cross-cultural issues don't come into play when child-rearing practices are similar. Or if people choose to give their children a cross-cultural or multicultural experience, that's a different matter. However, the potential for conflict exists when there is no element of choice, and a person of one culture cares for children of another culture whose value system is very different.

Some parents have choices and can find someone to care for their children who is in tune with their culture or in tune with their desires for a multicultural experience. However, parents must often take the only open slot in a subsidized child care center. In that case, there may be real trouble if the staff's ideas about good child care practices differ drastically from their own.

So it is important for teachers and caregivers who work with families whose culture differs from their own to take a good long look at where the parents are coming from when differences arise over issues of dependence and independence, feeding, toileting, napping, holding, comforting, "spoiling," discipline, and setting up the environment for play. Perhaps the teachers' or caregivers' attitudes will not change, but if they can at least hear what the parents have to say and be open to some negotiation, everyone is bound to benefit.[2] Of course, there will be some practices a particular teacher or caregiver won't bend on, but there may be others on which he or she will, after discussion. Other practices may conflict with licensing requirements, and that makes for even more discussion. Listen, look, be open, and try to understand.

LEARNING TO COMMUNICATE ACROSS CULTURES

I can't emphasize enough the importance of educating yourself when dealing with a person of a culture different from your own. I don't mean read books, though that may help. I do mean observe closely. You need to learn to communicate, even when you share a common language. Cross-cultural communication skills can be learned. Listed below are five areas of nonverbal communication where miscommunication can easily occur.

Personal Space

The place to start in learning to communicate across cultures is to become aware of proxemics, how close to stand or sit when communicating. We each have an invisible circle that surrounds us called "personal space." The size of the circle is to a great extent culturally determined. White Anglo- or European-Americans usually have about an arm's length of personal space surrounding them. That means when another mainstream culture American who is not an intimate approaches to talk, he or she automatically stops at the edge of the invisible circle. Some cultures have less personal space—smaller invisible circles; therefore some people stand closer to talk. They invade the white Anglo- or European-American's space without realizing it. In this situation, the invaded person feels uncomfortable and reacts by backing away, perhaps without even realizing it. The invader (who, of course, doesn't realizing he or she is invading) sees this retreating person as being distant or cold and is in turn seen as a "pushy" person, or perhaps just weird and suspect.

I once directed a workshop on cultural differences in which I conducted an exercise involving personal space. I had people walk around the room, stopping only to talk with each other—like at a cocktail party. It didn't take long to see that most of the people in the room stood at arm's length when talking to each other. One woman stood closer. Afterwards, we talked about personal space. This woman explained that she's a very friendly person who feels "unfriendly" if she stands at arm's length from someone. As it turned out, she was the only one in the room from another country. However, she didn't think her habit of standing close was culturally connected. That's how invisible culture can be.

Smiling

Smiling, touch, and eye contact are other communication skills specific to each culture. For example, Russians are reported to smile only when they are happy, not to be friendly. The friendly smile of some Canadians and Americans makes them feel as if those individuals are either fake or not too intelligent, whereas the Canadian and American interpret the nonsmiling behavior of the Russian as unfriendly. The Russian, who may be feeling very friendly indeed, would be shocked to know that he or she is being labeled the opposite.

For the Vietnamese, smiling has a variety of meanings.

> Almost anyone who has visited Vietnam or come in contact with the Vietnamese has noticed...a perpetual and enigmatic smile in all circumstances, unhappy as well as happy....Many foreign teachers in Vietnam have been irritated and frustrated when Vietnamese students smile in what appears to be the wrong time and place. They cannot understand how the students can smile when reprimanded, when not understanding the lessons being explained, and especially when they should have given an answer to the question instead of sitting still and smiling quietly. These teachers often thought the students were not only stupid and disobedient, but insolent as well. One thing they did not understand was that the students often smiled to show their teachers that they did not mind being reprimanded, or that they were indeed stupid for not being able to understand the lesson. Smiling at all times and places is a common characteristic of Vietnamese. There are, however, no guidelines to tell foreigners what meaning each smile represents in each situation...the Vietnamese smile may mean almost anything.[3]

Eye Contact

Find out about eye contact and respect. Is it important to look people in the eye or to look away when you talk to them? When cultures have the same patterns of eye contact, people feel comfortable with each other. But sometimes a person of one culture thinks a person who converses while looking away is shifty and dishonest, even though that person may think he or she is conveying respect. According to Root, Ho, and Sue, "Eye contact in the western culture is considered as an indication of attentiveness, although in the Asian culture, it may be viewed as a sign of lack of respect or deference."[4]

Some people feel uncomfortable under a steady gaze. Staring at someone, even while listening to him or her speak, may be considered rude. Lou Matheson says of Native Americans, "in most tribes staring is considered rude, and in some, prolonged eye contact is extremely disrespectful."[5]

Young discusses eye contact among black people and between blacks and whites. She says that many black families communicate better in ways other than words, one of which is deep eye contact.

> When parents want to impress something on a child, they give a deep long look. Black people often avoid eye contact with white people, giving the appearance of rudeness, since they don't seem to be paying attention. It may be, however, that they consider it disrespectful to look an authority figure in the eye. Or perhaps the eye contact, that goes with the words in white cultures brings too strong a communication to the black who regards it as more important than words.[6]

Staring at someone may even be considered harmful. Some cultures have the concept of "evil eye" in which prolonged intense staring can hurt the person being stared at.

Touch

Find out about touch, too. Is touching a sign of warmth and friendliness, is it an insult, or is it dangerous? In Vietnamese culture, touching people on the head robs them of their soul.[7]

Sometimes touching is a means of establishing or reflecting status. For example, in mainstream Canadian and American culture, bosses touch their secretaries much more often than secretaries touch their bosses.

When minor cultural rules about touch are broken, something just doesn't feel right. If a person is touched by the wrong person or in the wrong place, it can give misleading messages or feel uncomfortable. Consider the unwritten rules that white, mainstream, Canadian and American culture have about touching on the head. Anyone who touches someone else on the head is superior in some way—only inferiors (or intimates) are touched on the head.

Time Concepts

You'll get along with staff and parents of different cultures better if you find out the concept each has of time. Some cultures are more "now" oriented than others. White European- or Anglo-Americans are famous for being future oriented. In practical terms, this means differences in the concept of being "on time" as well as *planning* activities versus living in the moment.[8] Some parents consistently arrive late for scheduled meetings. This habit may be a personal idiosyncracy; but it can also mean that the parents have a different view of time. What does a deadline represent to them? This meaning can be related to cultural differences.

According to Edward T. Hall,

> Time is treated as a language, as a primary organizer for all activities, a synthesizer and integrator, a way of handling priorities and categorizing experience, a feedback mechanism for how things are going....Time is a core system of cultural, social, and personal life. In fact, nothing occurs except in some kind of time frame. A complicating factor in intercultural relations is that each culture has its own time frames in which the patterns are unique.[9]

If time is a language, as Hall says, timing is important to communication. For example, some people often talk around the subject—that's culturally appropriate. Others are more apt to regard "getting to the point" an immediate priority. It's not just a difference in personalities; it's a difference in cultures.[10] If you're trying to communicate with a parent, this piece of information could be vital.

THE INFLUENCE OF TEACHERS' AND CAREGIVERS' ATTITUDES ON THEIR LEARNING

It is beyond the scope of this book to give you the details of every culture you might encounter as a teacher or caregiver in this country. However, the Further Reading section and the bibliography will direct you to where to get the information. Still, it is asking a lot of someone who works long hours at caregiving to spend more long hours doing homework.

I suggest that you learn about each culture from the parents in your program. Start by creating an intake questionnaire that asks for cultural information. Ask questions such as, What is the primary language spoken at home by the father? By the mother? Ask how the parents describe their child's ethnicity. Find out who else lives in the home. See if you can open up some doors to communication by showing interest in cultural matters. You can also study on the spot—learning culture by observing yourself and the people you interact with in your program.

Become aware of your discomforts and discuss them when appropriate. Encourage others to develop this same awareness. When you begin to share, you'll learn more than you could learn from any book. You gain the most meaningful information from real people of the culture you are learning about.

You learn about cultural conflicts by being aware of what you are feeling and trying to put yourself in the shoes of the other person to understand what he or she might be feeling. You learn about true differences in caregiving and child-rearing practices best from people who practice them rather than secondhand through lectures and readings.

Many teachers and caregivers can easily do this firsthand learning because of the cultural diversity of the parents in their programs. To what extent they seize the opportunity depends on their attitudes and openness. I see a progression of attitudes toward differences from awareness, tolerance, and acceptance to respect and appreciation. Beyond that lie celebration, support, and finally using differences as resources to expand and enrich one's own life.

FOR FURTHER READING

Anderson, P. "Explaining Intercultural Differences in Nonverbal Communication," in L. Samovar and R. Porter, (eds), *Intercultural Communication: A Reader.* Belmont, Calif.: Wadsworth, 1994. Helps clarify some of the difficulty behind cross-cultural communication.

Gudykunst, W. BV., ed. *Intercultural Communication Theory: Current Perspectives.* Beverly Hills: Sage, 1983. A look at communication theory as it relates to cross-cultural exchanges.

Delpit, Lisa. "The Silenced Dialogue: Power and Pedagogy in Educating Other People's Children," *Harvard Educational Review*, 58(8) 1988, pp. 280–298. Gives a perspective on why cross-cultural communication is so important.

Derman-Sparks, Louise, "The Process of Culturally Sensitive Care," in *Infant/Toddler Caregiving: A Guide to Culturally Sensitive Care*, Peter Mangione, ed., Sacramento, Calif.: Far West Laboratory and California Department of Education, 1995. Gives some specific ideas regarding what to do in a cross-cultural situation.

NOTES

1. Lally, J. Ronald. "The Impact on Child Care Policies and Practices on Infant/Toddler Identity Formation," *Young Children*, 51(1), November 1995, pp. 58–67.

2. There are many instances where parent and teachers come from the same culture but have differing values, ideas, beliefs, and practices. Teachers must respect these parents even though they do not share the same views on many subjects. It is sometimes eas-

ier to understand and explain differences when a cultural label can be attached to them. It's harder to accept and respect diversity when the person looks like us. It is also important not to make assumptions about people's culture based on their appearance. I learned that lesson when, as a preschool teacher, I met a redhaired, freckled child who I assumed was Anglo-American. However, to my surprise, the child was Mexican and didn't speak a word of English. I learned this lesson again when, at a training conference in Hawaii for child care, we went around the room and stated our background and ethnicity. The ethnicity of many of the people didn't match my first assumptions. I learned that you can't determine the ethnicity of people based on how they look.

3. Duong Thanh Binh, *A Handbook for Teachers of Vietnamese Students: Hints for Dealing with Cultural Differences in Schools.* Arlington, Vir.: Center for Applied Linguistics, 1975, p. 18.

4. Root, Maria, Ho, Christine, and Sue, Stanley, "Issues in the Training of Counselors for Asian Americans," in *Cross-Cultural Training for Mental Health Professionals,* H. Lefley and P. Pedersen, eds. Springfield, Ill.: Charles C. Thomas, 1986, p. 202.

5. Matheson, Lou, "If You Are Not an Indian, How Do You Treat an Indian?" in Lefley and Pedersen, *Cross-Cultural Training,* p. 124.

   According to Morrow, while talking, Vietnamese, Cambodian, and Laotian people do not look steadily at a respected person's eyes. Morrow, Robert D., "Cultural Differences—Be Aware!" *Academic Therapy* 23(2), November 1987, p. 147.

6. Young, V. H., "Family and Childhood in a Southern Georgia Community," *American Anthropologist* 72, 1970, p. 270.

7. Duong, *A Handbook for Teachers of Vietnamese Students.*

8. Lefley and Pedersen, *Cross-Cultural Training for Mental Health Professionals.*

9. Hall, E. T., *The Dance of Life, the other Dimension of Time.* New York: Anchor Press, 1984, p. 3.

10. Ibid.

    According to Morrow, the Vietnamese, Cambodians, and Laotians prefer to talk around a subject before coming to the point rather than talking about it directly. Morrow, "Cultural Differences," p. 148.

    According to Hall, in some cultures, a person with something on his or her mind will talk all around the point instead of letting the person being addressed know what's bothering him or her. It's expected that the person will know and will make the point himself or herself. Hall, Edward T., *Beyond Culture.* Garden City, N.Y.: Anchor Press/Doubleday, 1981, p. 112.

    According to Root, Ho, and Sue, "The Western emphasis on directness in speech may alienate many Asians. Indirectness in speech is preferred since it avoids direct confrontation which may cause loss of face." Root, Ho, and Sue, "Issues in the Training of Counselors," p. 202.

CHAPTER THREE

Toilet Training: An Example of a Cultural Conflict

All human relationships are bound to bring conflicts and disagreements. Parent–caregiver relationships exemplify this principle very well. When the parent is of one culture and the caregiver of another, the possibility of conflict multiplies.

Although cultural conflicts can create quite a challenge, in many ways, they are an asset. You can not only gain strength and skills as you work your way through them, but you can gain new knowledge as well. What follows is an example of a cultural conflict. I picked one to start with that is heavily laden with emotion for most people, one in which there is no obvious solution.

> Here's the conflict scene. A mother and a caregiver are engaged in an intense discussion. "I just can't do what you want," says the caregiver. "I don't have time with all these other children to care for. Besides," she adds hesitantly, "I don't believe in toilet training a one year old."
>
> "But she's already trained!" the mother says emphatically. "All you have to do is put her on the potty."
>
> "She's not trained—you're trained." The caregiver's voice is still calm and steady, but a red flush is beginning to creep up her neck toward her face.
>
> "You just don't understand!" The mother picks up her daughter and diaper bag and sweeps out the door.
>
> "No, *you're* the one who doesn't understand" mutters the caregiver, busying herself with a pile of dirty dishes precariously stacked on the counter.

Both caregiver and mother are correct. Neither understands the other. They are embroiled in a cultural conflict.[1] Unfortunately, the conversation ended before they could begin to do some problem solving around their misunderstandings. If they had continued to talk, they *might* have eventually begun to see each other's point of view. Somewhere down the road they might even have reached an agreement that both could live with.

What is "cultural" about this argument? Unless your experience is otherwise, bowel and bladder control seem to be biological facts rather than cultural differences. It is hard to justify toilet training a one year old when research points to a later start at toilet training.[2]

CONFLICTING DEFINITIONS AND GOALS

Part of the problem of the conflict resides in the definition and goal of toilet training. If the caregiver defines toilet training as teaching or encouraging the child independently to take care of his or her own toileting needs and her goal is to accomplish this as quickly and painlessly as possible, she'll regard twelve months as too early to start. Children of twelve months need adult help. However, if toilet training is regarded as a reduction of diapers and the method is to form a partnership with the child to do just that, you'll start as soon as you can read the children's signals and "catch them in time." In the first case, the focus is on independence, in the second, on interdependence or mutual dependence.[3]

How is such a partnership between adult and child possible, you may ask. Here's what Janice Hale-Benson says:

> Because Black babies are held so much of the time, there is an immediate response to urination and bowel movements. Hence from an early age, there is an association in the infant's mind between these functions, and action from the mother. Consequently, when the mother seeks to toilet train the child (in the early and stringent manner that has been observed in the Black community), the child is accustomed to her direct involvement in the process. In contrast, the transition is more startling for middle-class American infants whose functions typically occur alone. The mother begins to interfere with bowel and bladder activity after many months of only cursory attention. There is greater continuity, then, in the behavior of Black mothers.[4]

Here's what Dorothy Lee says:

> American observers had noticed that Chinese babies had learned, by the time they were about six months old, to indicate that they wanted to micturate; yet they seemed to be treated very permissively with no attempt at toilet training....When the baby wants to urinate, his whole body participates in the preliminary process. The Chinese mother, holding the baby in her arms, learns to be sensitive to the minute details of this process, and to hold her baby away from herself at exactly the critical moment. Eventually, the infant learns to ask to be held out. The mother neither tries to control the baby, nor does she train the infant to control himself according to imposed standards. Instead, she sensitizes herself to his rhythm, and helps him to adopt social

discipline with spontaneity, starting from his unique pattern. What is interesting here is that as an end result of this, the baby is "toilet-trained" at a very early age; but it has been an experience of spontaneity for him and his autonomy has remained inviolate, because his mother has had the sensitivity and the patience to "listen" to him.[5]

I'm not suggesting that a caregiver's goal should be the constant holding involved in either of these approaches to toilet training. I'm merely suggesting that caregivers should do what they can to prolong the discussion when a parent has that goal. If the mother doesn't stomp out the door, she'll probably eventually see the realities of day care and come to understand the caregiver's goal and reasons for the later start. In addition, the caregiver will learn more about cultural differences. He or she may even learn something new about human behavior and child development!

AN EXAMPLE OF BETTER CAREGIVER-PARENT COMMUNICATION

Here's a replay of that scene showing the caregiver trying to prolong the discussion by acknowledging the parent's strong feelings.

"I see you have strong feelings about my continuing what you are doing at home. I'm sorry, but I just can't do what you want," says the caregiver. "I don't have time with all these other children to care for. But I can see how much you want me to."

"Yes, I do want you to. It's important to me that my daughter wear dry clothes all the time—and it's so easy if you just put her on the potty when she has to go. Then I won't have all those diapers at home."

"I can tell this is really important to you…"

"It sure is! I just don't understand why you want to keep changing diapers when you don't have to."

"I guess the problem is you and I have different ideas about toilet training."

"Yes, it seems we do."

The chances of the two reaching some sort of agreement in just one short conversation are slim. However, the door is open for further conversations about this subject because instead of arguing and setting up blocks, the caregiver tried to keep communication going.

It's often hard for parents to explain their points of view in the face of knowledgeable caregivers who carry an aura of expertise. It becomes even harder with parents who do not speak English fluently.

The previous dialogue got the problem out on the table, and although the two didn't reach any agreements or conclusions, they both discussed the issue in a direct way. However, some cultures avoid the direct approach. Laying out the problem in a forthright manner is an insult to the listener. According to Hall, in some cultures, a person with something on his or her mind will "expect his interlocutor to know what's bothering him, so that he doesn't have to be specific. The result is that he will talk around and around the point, in effect putting all the pieces in place except the crucial one. Placing it properly—this keystone—is the role of his interlocutor. To do this for him is an insult."[6] This may seem very strange to those who don't argue in this way, but it is right and normal to those who do. Direct ways of stating problems are strange, if not insulting.

Even if the parent in the example had been able to convey the problem effectively, even if she had been able to make the caregiver understand how important it is that her daughter be given the kind of attention needed to remain dry most of the time, that doesn't resolve the conflict. It's not just the understanding that's important, though in some exchanges that's the first and most difficult obstacle to overcome.

Once he or she understands the problem, the caregiver must decide how to respond. In this case, it is unlikely that the caregiver would have agreed to go along with the mother, no matter how sensitive or understanding she was. Infant/caregiver ratios don't allow constant holding of a single child. Besides, if the caregiver didn't believe in interdependence, should she do something against her own value system just because a parent wants her to?

This is a difficult situation. There are many questions to be asked and no right answers to any of them. As a caregiver, you must consider the child's needs, the parent's needs and values, your own needs and values, and the program's philosophy. If you are clear about your own view and that view is in tune with the program's philosophy, you stand on solid ground. People who are unclear or uncertain are more likely to be defensive and staunchly defend their own side without considering the other person's side. If you're secure, you'll have an easier time truly listening to a parent and understanding her child. With an awareness and understanding of the elements of this conflict, you'll be able to create a relationship and eventually an ongoing dialogue.

FOUR OUTCOMES TO CULTURAL CONFLICTS

I see four possible outcomes to working toward resolving cultural conflicts. Let's look at how each outcome might play out in a particular situation. For example, an eighteen month old child, whose mother says is toilet trained, arrives in day care without diapers. She wets her pants repeatedly, using up her spare clothes and the extra clothes of the center. This situation has the potential to become a conflict between parent and staff, if it happens more than once. What are the possible outcomes of this conflict?

Resolution Through Negotiation

If both the parent and caregiver can work together and problem solve this issue, they may find a mutually satisfying solution. "Let's figure this out together," is a good way to start the discussion. If they come to a joint agreement that involves action by both, they've resolved the problem through negotiation. For example, the mother could say, "I'll continue to toilet train my child at home, but will bring her to the center in diapers." And the caregiver might say, "I'll try each day to put her on the toilet when I have enough staff and it will work out."

Ongoing Management of the Unresolved Conflict

The caregiver may disagree with the mother's idea that the child is ready for toilet training but may be unable to convince the mother that she's wrong. In this case, the conflict may continue in a negative way with smoldering tensions and continual arguments that both will have to cope with or in a positive way with both managing the conflict by agreeing to disagree. Trust can make a big difference as to whether the ongoing management of a conflict is negative or positive. It helps if the caregiver knows that the parent loves the child. Indeed, some caregivers believe that all parents love their children and that they are doing the best they can with what they know, who they are, and the circumstances they find themselves in. On the other hand, for a parent, trust comes when he or she knows that a caregiver has the child's best interests at heart. This kind of trust helps adults agree to disagree.

Teacher Education

Suppose that the caregiver learns from the parent how to keep the child dry. In that case, the caregiver learns the parent's way, which helps broaden the caregiver's view of child care practices. When teachers understand the parent's point of view, they may broaden, adjust, or fine tune their own goals, policies, or procedures to be more like the parent's.

Parent Education

Perhaps the teacher convinces the parent that the child isn't ready to be trained because she wets all the time. She may also show how hard it is on the child to be continually taken away from what she's doing to have her wet clothes changed. Parent education is fine as long as the teacher is sensitive to parental goals and values. It's not good to alienate parents from their own cultural beliefs and practices.

SHOULD TEACHERS EVER CONVINCE PARENTS TO CHANGE?

This question is hard to answer because the goals of the parents must be considered. Do the parents want themselves or their children to be "Americanized?" Perhaps they will return to their own country and their concern is whether their children will still fit into their own culture. This is a legitimate concern.

For families who are already Canadians or Americans but not in mainstream culture, the issue of retaining their own cultural practices is important. If we are to have a salad bowl instead of a melting pot, diversity must be honored and preserved so that each group keeps its own flavor.

However, flavors change. Culture is never static; it continues to evolve. Further, when one culture rubs up against another, both are transformed. A challenge for many parents in this country is to maintain their cultural identity and pass it on to their children in the face of this inevitable evolution. This need for retaining cultural identity can become a tremendous source of internal conflict when members of a culture perceive that they are held back from full participation in society because of cultural behaviors, values, or goals. If you have never experienced that conflict yourself, try to imagine the tremendous strain it would cause in you if you were faced with the problem.

PARENT EDUCATION AND TEACHER-CAREGIVER EDUCATION

I do believe in parent education, even when it creates conflicts in people of diverse cultures. However, I also believe in teacher-caregiver education. No matter how well versed you are in developmentally appropriate practices, you must realize that even child development information based on sound research is culturally biased. Researchers have values. They consider questions important to their culture. They look at results through cultural spectacles. For example, researchers, recognizing that a certain kind of langauge background is related to school success, find deficiencies in children who come from a different kind of language background. When researchers examine the issue from the cultural perspective of the families of these children, they can see strengths in the differences.

I'm not saying to throw out child development information. I am saying that we all have something to learn from taking a culturally sensitive perspective.

Most of us also need to learn not to judge other cultures with our own yardsticks. People tend to be ethnocentric, that is, to see their own culture as "normal" and others as "not normal." Most feel that their own culture is superior—that's natural. Recognize and accept that fact in yourself and others. At the same time, understand that all cultures have evolved to the way they are for specific reasons. Cultures aren't superior or inferior; they just *are*.

Knowing all this, how do you manage to survive conflicts with parents? How do you come out with your own cultural beliefs intact while helping the parents feel good about themselves and their culture? And how do you even have these discussions about issues when most of your time is taken up with meeting the needs of a group of children? It isn't easy. It takes a good deal of willingness and a lot of patience plus communication and problem-solving skills. It helps to be well grounded in child development theory as well.

SUGGESTIONS FOR APPROACHING CULTURAL CONFLICTS

Here is a summary of hints to help you deal with the cultural conflicts that can arise in a child care setting:

1. Take it slow. Don't expect to resolve each conflict immediately. Building understandings and relationships takes time. As already stated, some conflicts won't be resolved; they'll just be managed. You have to learn to cope with differences when there is no common meeting ground or resolution. This coping sounds hard, but it's possible, if you're willing to accept the fact that resolution is not always the outcome of disputes.

2. Understand yourself. Become clear about your own values and goals. Know what you believe in. Have a bottom line, but leave space above it to be flexible.

3. Become sensitive to your own discomfort. Tune in on those times when something bothers you instead of just ignoring it and hoping it will go away. Work to identify what specific behaviors of others make you uncomfortable. Try to discover exactly what in yourself creates this discomfort.

4. Learn about other cultures. Books, classes, and workshops help, but watch for stereotypes and biased information. Your best source of information comes from the parents in your program. Check out what they believe about their cultures, and see if it fits with other information you receive. However, don't ever make one person a representative of his or her culture. Listen to individuals, take in the information they give you, but don't generalize to whole cultures. Keep your mind open as you learn. Check out your point of view. There's a difference between finding and celebrating diversity versus explaining deficiencies.

5. Find out what the parents in your program, individually, want for their children. What are their goals? What are their caregiving practices?

What concerns do they have about their child in your program? Encourage them to talk to you. Encourage them to ask questions. You may find out about cultures this way, or you may just find out about individual or familial differences. All are important.

6. Be a risk taker. If you are secure enough, you may feel you can afford to make mistakes. Mistakes are a part of cross-cultural communication. It helps to have a good support system behind you when you take risks and make mistakes. Ask questions, investigate assumptions, confess your curiosity—but do it all as respectfully as possible.

7. Communicate, dialogue, negotiate. If you have a chance to build a relationship before getting into negotiations, you're more likely eventually to reach a mutually satisfying point. You'll find examples of the communication, dialogue, negotiation process throughout this book.

8. Share power. Empowerment is an important factor in the dialogue-negotiation process. Although some see empowerment (allowing others to experience their own personal power) as threatening, in reality, empowerment creates new forms of power. Some teachers and care-givers fear that empowerment means giving away their own power, but this is not true! No one can give personal power, and no one can take it away. We all have our personal power, though we can be discouraged or prevented from recognizing or using it. Sharing power, or empowerment, enhances everyone's power.

In conclusion, hard as it may be to take the risks involved in cross-cultural encounters, to learn what is needed to understand culturally different people, to gain skills in communication, and to cope when conflicts arise, exposure to more than one culture is a definite asset. As you care for children from various cultural backgrounds, everyone gains. You, the children, and the parents have the opportunity to learn more about and appreciate human diversity.

FOR FURTHER READING

Derman-Sparks, Louise, "The Process of Culturally Sensitive Care," in *Infant/Toddler Caregiving: A Guide to Culturally Sensitive Care*, Mangione, Peter, ed., Sacramento, Calif.: Far West Laboratory and California Department of Education, 1995. A how-to guide for negotiating cultural differences.

Fisher, Roger, and Ury, William, *Getting to Yes: Negotiating Agreement Without Giving In.* New York: Penguin Books, 1991. Helps with the negotiation process.

Gonzalez-Mena, Janet, "Taking A Culturally Sensitive Approach in Infant-Toddler Programs," *Young Children* 47(2), January 1992, 4–9. More information about cultural conflicts.

Gonzalez-Mena, Janet, and Stonehouse, Anne, "In the Child's Best Interests," *Child Care Information Exchange* 106, November 1995, 17–20. A broader look at what the "child's best interests" really means.

NOTES

1. This particular issue doesn't have to be a cultural conflict; it can be a generational conflict. My own mother often bragged to me that I was toilet trained at a year. She used to call me a lazy mother because I was relaxed about training my own children, who were over two before they exhibited the signs of readiness I was looking for. But I had research and a whole pediatric and early childhood community to back me up, so I stuck to my guns. We never did see eye to eye on this issue. It wasn't until I ran into the same issue as a cultural conflict that I began to be able to see it from a different perspective.

2. Brazelton, T. B., "A Child Oriented Approach to Toilet Training," *Pediatrics* 29(1), January 1962, pp. 121–128.

3. "Americans, who value independence and individuality, see the baby as dependent, undifferentiated...the Japanese, who prize close interdependence between child and adult, regard the infant as having a small component of autonomy...believe they must tempt the infant into a dependent role, rush to soothe a crying infant, respond quietly to the baby's excited babbling, and sleep with the young child at night in order to encourage the mutual bonding necessary for adult life." Kagan, Jerome, *The Nature of the Child*. New York: Basic Books, 1984, p. 29.

4. Hale-Benson, Janice, "Black Children: Their Roots, Culture, and Learning Styles," in *Understanding the Multicultural Experience in Early Childhood Education*, Olivia N. Saracho and Bernard Spodek, eds. Washington, D.C.: National Association for the Education of Young Children, 1983, p. 24.

5. Lee, Dorothy, *Freedom and Culture*. Englewood Cliffs, N.J.: Prentice-Hall, 1959, p. 8.

6. Hall, Edward T., *Beyond Culture*. Garden City, N.Y.: Anchor Press/Doubleday, 1981, p. 112.

CHAPTER FOUR

Caregiving Routines: Feeding and Sleeping

I n the beginning of life, the processes of taking in food and going to sleep are quite intertwined. As the child grows older, they become separated, though to what extent and how soon depend on the adult attitudes toward the two.

EATING AND SLEEPING: TWO CONTRASTING PATTERNS

Pattern One: Schedules

Two patterns emerge when looking at adult approaches related to babies eating and sleeping. One pattern is a movement toward a schedule—toward consistency. The goal is to get the baby in a routine so that eating and sleeping become regular and predictable. This is done by regulating the feedings and keeping the baby awake at certain times during the day or in the evening.

The schedule may not start from day one, but from day one the parents or caregivers in this pattern are trying to get the baby to distinguish between day and night. The goal is to get the baby to sleep longer and longer periods at night and spend waking and eating time during the day.

The baby may be fed at first according to need—that is, whenever the adult thinks he or she is hungry; however, eventually some sort of a schedule establishes itself, and the adults concerned feel a sense of accomplishment. The baby takes a bottle or is breast-fed every three or four hours and catnaps periodically between feedings, sleeping six to eight hours at night. The next step comes when the baby settles into a schedule that includes three meals and two naps a day. As time goes on, the morning nap gets later and later until it blends with the afternoon nap, and the adult announces, "She's down to one nap a day now."

Babies who are raised by routine-loving adults usually have a specific bedtime as well as regular feeding and nap times. Things that change the routine may be upsetting to adults and babies alike, and the adult may explain fussiness as a disruption of routine: "she's fussy because she didn't get her nap today" or "he's fussy because his schedule's all off."

These adults believe that establishing a routine, a schedule, creates a daily rhythm, a sameness that is important to good health and happiness. "Easy babies" are those who adjust to routines. "Hard babies" are those who defy the adult's attempts to schedule and regulate them.

Pattern Two: Natural Rhythms

Some adults don't go by the clock; they don't have schedules. Their own lives may be in tune with their natural body rhythms, and if they can resist the takeover of their lives by the clock, they do so. Even if they can't resist for themselves, they may be dedicated to the idea of doing it for babies.

The natural rhythm pattern of sleep is linked at the beginning to feeding rhythms. Pattern two works best with breast-feeding because the milk is always ready and the right temperature, and adults don't think in terms of ounces consumed. Mothers who sleep with their babies and breast-feed upon need are less likely to be concerned about how soon the baby sleeps through the night. True pattern two people feed when the baby seems to be hungry without regard to how long it's been since the last feeding. (This is a contrast to pattern one feeders, who make statements like, "He drank six ounces just two hours ago; he can't possibly be starving now.") Because the amount of breast milk consumed isn't measured, the pattern two person is less apt to be convinced the baby isn't hungry when crying.

An Example of the Two Patterns

Contrast the difference. Pretend you're the pattern one mother of a two month old. You went to bed late because you were watching a good movie on TV and because you wanted to get a last feeding in so *maybe* your son would sleep through the night for a change. You woke him up at 11 P.M. to feed him, and he went right back to sleep. Now you're asleep yourself and enjoying a pleasant dream, when from the other room comes a dreadful howl.

"Maybe he'll go back to sleep," you think to yourself as you open one eye and look at the clock, which announces 3 A.M. in glowing red digits.

He doesn't go back to sleep. He howls louder. You drag yourself out of bed, reassuring him in your kindest voice that you are coming. Pulling on your bathrobe, you head for the kitchen. The floor is cold on your bare feet. You blink at the bright light from the refrigerator and are startled to see emptiness inside. Where is the bottle you prepared for this event? Gone. You remember then that you used the last one at the 11 P.M. feeding.

So you start making a bottle. It seems to take forever. The cries from the other room urge you to hurry. Finally, you emerge from the kitchen, bottle in hand.

You sleepily change your son, who howls throughout the ordeal. Finally, the two of you are settled in the rocking chair in his room. He sucks frantically at first, clawing at your hand with his tiny fingers, but slows down as the worst of the hunger pangs subside.

An hour later you finally slip back into your bed, your cold feet finding little comfort between the now chilly sheets. You turn over and close your eyes, but sleep won't come. You're just too wide awake. You lie in the dark, listening to the little contented noises coming from your son's room, and you think about all the sleepless nights you've spent in the last two months.

Now pretend you're the same mother in the same situation, but you're a pattern two person. Contrast that scene to this one.

You watched the movie in bed, your son snuggled beside you, already asleep. You didn't wake him at 11 o'clock for a feeding because you know he'll wake when he is hungry. When the movie was over, you turned off the light, rolled over, and went to sleep. You wake sometime in the night to the movement of your son, who is making soft sounds. You don't turn on the light or look at the clock; you roll over, get rid of the clothing between you, and help him in his search for your nipple. He finds it without either of you being fully awake. He sucks vigorously. You doze off. When you wake in the morning, you're not sure how many times he ate in the night, nor does it seem important to you. You know that he eats when he's hungry.

What happens when pattern two babies (natural rhythms, ignore the clock) go into a day-care program that's structured for pattern one schedule types?

Pattern one and pattern two in child care programs   Usually pattern clashes don't create a problem with younger babies because they often are encouraged to follow their own schedule or natural rhythms for both feeding and sleep. However, the goal for even young babies may be to establish an individual daily schedule if pattern one caregivers are part of the staff.

Feeding for young babies is usually an individual matter, though no one is there to breast-feed whenever the baby is hungry, so the individual natural feeding rhythms won't work in quite the same way even if the caregiver firmly believes in them. Sometimes a caregiver will try to duplicate the natural rhythms approach using a bottle and ignoring the clock. But if the baby wants to eat very often, the caregiver who complies may meet with disapproval from those who feel constant feeding isn't good for babies and that bottles should be spaced, even if no schedule is intended. A difference between breast-feeding and bottle-feeding, as mentioned before, is that adults know how much bottle-fed babies have consumed.

For young babies, the most common approach in child care is to encourage an individual schedule for eating and sleeping, taking each baby's needs into consideration. As the babies grow older, some attempt is usually made to coordinate all the children's schedules until by two or sometimes by three years of age, all or most eat and sleep according to the same schedule.

The issue of sleeping alone   The issue of sleeping alone in a crib sometimes arises in child care. A pattern one parent is more likely to put her baby to sleep in another room, or at least in his own crib in her room. She is most likely to regard her baby as an individual who needs to come to see himself as separate from her.[1]

A pattern two parent may also have a crib but may not use it as much as the pattern one parent. Some pattern two parents never even buy a crib, preferring that their babies not sleep alone.[2] Pattern one and pattern two people may disapprove of each other. Each has strong reasons why the other is wrong.

Most programs in Canada and the United States lean more toward pattern one than pattern two and are dedicated to the idea that each child needs a crib to sleep in; indeed, there is often a licensing regulation to back up the program's policy.

Here's what happened in one program. A Southeast Asian immigrant family enrolled their baby in an infant center program. The baby had never slept by himself before, and when he was put into a crib off in a quiet, darkened room, he got very upset. It wasn't just the ordinary upset of a child who was resisting going to sleep even though tired; it was a panic reaction of a child who was very fearful of the situation. No matter what the staff tried to do to help this child sleep alone, nothing worked. He would sleep only near someone in the midst of the activity of the playroom. Being by himself to sleep was a fearful and foreign situation for him.

The staff wanted to accommodate the child's special need, which they perceived to be a cultural difference; however, state licensing regulations got in the way. But this story has a happy ending! The staff was able to convince the licensing authority to grant a waiver to the regulation that infants sleep alone in a crib in a room separate from the play area.

Putting children to sleep   Adults, even within the same culture, don't necessarily agree about ways to put children to sleep. Some feel it is important for babies to discover their own soothing devices and use them to settle down to sleep. These adults are likely to put the tired baby into a crib and let him put himself to sleep, even if he creates a fuss before he finally settles down.

Other adults use their own soothing devices to put the baby to sleep and are not willing for babies to be unhappy if they can help it. Sometimes this attitude is influenced by culture; other times it relates to living circumstances (when a crying baby disturbs others, adults may keep that baby from crying out of respect). Imagine a situation where a number of people live in a small apartment and a baby who puts himself to sleep by crying hard every night for fifteen minutes moves in. Respect for the adults' peace and quiet may have priority over the baby's method of putting himself to sleep.

Putting older children to sleep is another issue because if they don't sleep in cribs, or do sleep in cribs but climb out of them, you either have to find some way to put them down and keep them there so they can put themselves to sleep, or you have to use various means to settle them down and put them to sleep. If you're a dedicated pattern one person, you may train them to stay on their cot or blanket or in their crib long enough so they fall asleep either on schedule or when you perceive they are tired. If you are a pattern two person, you may be inclined to be less firm about "putting the child down," but you may expect children to "put themselves down" whenever they are tired.

Very few teachers or caregivers in my experience use this latter approach, partly because the adults need a break from the children, and they get it at nap time. Indeed, even if they wanted to let children rest whenever they wanted rather than according to schedule, they'd find various kinds of outside pressures to create a regular "nap time" in their program. They'd also get arguments about children being overtired and not able to put themselves down. A criticism of pattern two adults is that they let the children "go until they drop from exhaustion." The answer to that criticism is that children who are taught to tune in on their own body rhythms from the beginning are aware of their needs to rest just as they are aware of their needs to eat. Pattern two people believe that it's good training for adulthood to get in touch with one's own physical needs—especially in a society in which so many are out of touch.

FEEDING AND EATING

Both the sleeping and feeding processes are highly charged with feelings and have great potential for conflicts between teachers or caregivers and parents. The following scene shows an example of a cultural conflict.

A mother arrives to pick up her son from an infant center. She enters the room to find him seated, waving a spoon in the air with one hand while jamming mushy cereal into his already full mouth with the other one. The mother hurries over to him, frowning, and says gruffly to the caregiver sitting close by watching him, "Where's a washcloth?"

She takes the cloth handed to her, and as she briskly cleans up her protesting son, she is mumbling under her breath. The gist of her mumbling concerns her dissatisfaction with the self-feeding process and the mess created.

The caregiver, who is now cleaning up another child nearby, tries to talk about self-help skills and sensory experiences, but the angry mother's back is turned the whole time as she works over her son. She finally gets her child's hands and face clean, but his clothes, in spite of the bib, still show signs of the meal he has just enjoyed. Hurriedly she changes his shirt, which now clashes with the pants he has on. She looks at the outfit and shakes her head in disgust. She is still looking distressed as she bustles out the door, diaper bag and son in hand.

The caregiver, angry herself by now, sits down for a minute to cool off before dealing with the children needing her attention.

Dealing with a Conflict by Creating a Dialogue

A parent's attitude may trigger anger in the teacher or caregiver, which makes him or her less inclined to try to understand the parent's perspective. It hurts to feel attacked and criticized. However, it is vital that teachers and caregivers tune in on parents in conflicts like this—not just defensively write them off.

How can a teacher or caregiver communicate by creating a dialogue when parents leave like this one did? What do you do with angry parents who will neither talk nor listen?

Whatever you do, don't give up! Work hard to build a relationship. Don't be as concerned about getting your point of view across as about opening lines of communication. It helps if the parent feels you care about and respect her. One way to convey this caring and respect is to tune in on feelings. When you acknowledge how a parent feels, you have a better chance eventually to get to a dialogue.

Above all try not to get defensive about your own perspective. Try hard to tune in to the parent's point of view. Start by looking at goals and priorities. Are you on the same wavelength? In a situation like the previous one, you probably aren't. Whereas your priority may be self-help skills and sensory experiences at mealtimes, the parent may have much stronger feelings about neatness for a lot of different reasons.[3]

Varying Perspectives on Early Self-Feeding

The experts in this country agree that it is important to encourage babies to take part in the feeding process and hand it over completely soon after the baby can get the food from plate to mouth, no matter how much mess results. Comer and Poussaint say, "When your baby makes reasonably good attempts to feed himself, encourage it. Not only does this support a feeling of independence, but it also permits him to develop greater skill in using his hands."[4] Other experts advise leniency about letting children *touch*, and even *play with* their food, and even see these behaviors as *sensory experiences.*[5]

In some cultures, food is revered and is never considered a plaything, not at the eating table or at the activity table. Many people frown on such things as finger painting with pudding, playing with play dough, or placing beans or rice in a "sensory table." Anyone who has experienced severe food shortages may be horrified at the thought of playing with food. Some people, even without personal starvation experience, have strong feelings about world hunger. They feel that it's wrong to use food as a plaything.

The issue of food shortages may be combined with the cleanup issue. Anyone without washers or dryers and plenty of extra clothes may have a different attitude toward letting babies play with food or have a sensory experience. A family may have plenty of everything but live in a home not set up for messy meals. In both cases, the priority is on preventing rather than cleaning up messes. Prevention means spoon-feeding the baby.

Sodetaini-Shibata says this about the Japanese approach to self-feeding:

> Children are fed until they acquire the ability to handle a spoon on their own...but parents often resort to the use of both self-feeding and adult-feeding....As the child approaches school-age, feeding by the parents is weaned, and it is stopped when the child enters school....[O]rderliness and tidiness are highly stressed in the Japanese daily life.[6]

Valuing neatness may be less of an issue than lack of time. When parents have to rush to feed their babies and clean up after them, they may find it more expedient to continue to spoon-feed until their children can eat neatly and efficiently by themselves, which may be as late as four years old.

The opposing values of independence versus interdependence often lie behind conflicts that involve self-help skills, like self-feeding. I remember some of the Hispanic parents I used to work with who spoon-fed their children far beyond the age that I considered reasonable. I was trying to make their children independent through early self-help skills; they had different ideas. They were less concerned about children helping themselves than they were about teaching them to help others. By feeding them, they were modeling the behavior they were trying to teach. The goal was interdependence.

If you see little reason for children to stand alone (on their own two feet, as the expression goes) but lots of reasons for them to experience and value relationships, you may be very willing to let self-help skills come much later. You may see a value in one person being dependent on another. The point is mutual dependence. Now it's the small child dependent on more capable adults. Once that phase is over, other dependencies will take their place. But dependency isn't a one-way proposition as you grow up; just as you are dependent, so are you depended upon. Interdependency is a lifelong condition, one that relates to permanent attachment with one's family or one's people, something that is highly valued in some cultures.

Dietary Practices as a Factor in Conflict

What to eat brings the potential for more conflict. As an example, some parents have strong moral or religious reasons to be vegetarians. Others cite health reasons to avoid meat. Many cultures depend more on other foods than on meat for their nutritional requirements and don't regard meat as an important dietary factor. Often this is because meat is expensive and not readily available. Some Mexican and Chinese families, for example, use meat sparingly in a few dishes for flavoring rather than for the bulk of their nutrition, depending on legumes and grains for the mainstay food. (Beans, rice, chiles, and tortillas are standard fare for some Mexican tables, for example.) As a basic diet, this makes good sense, especially when compared to the excess of animal products in the greasy diet of many people in the United States today.

A teacher or caregiver accustomed to using meat only as flavoring is likely to be more understanding of a vegetarian parent than a teacher or caregiver who comes from an old-fashioned farm family and doesn't consider it a meal unless meat is served. Many variations of vegetarianism exist and it's important that teachers and caregivers understand each one. Strict vegetarians are very different from vegetarians who only have eliminated red meat from their diet.

It is critical to determine exactly what can and cannot be eaten. It may be helpful to know the reason for the family's vegetarian diet or for *any* type of specialized diet. Families with moral reasons are often not as strict as families with religious reasons. Find out what the prohibitions are and how strict they are. Staying kosher, for example, involves much more than just avoiding pork. If you are unaware that packaged foods contain a kosher mark, you might easily feed a child nonkosher food. Also, combinations of foods, such as meat and milk products, are to be avoided. Any religious group that has restrictions about pork has to avoid foods containing lard, such as some types of crackers, ice creams, and many other foods. And, diets may change with certain times of the year and particular holidays. This type of information must be received from the parents. If it's important to them, they'll probably offer the information. However, it's up to the teacher to take it seriously.

Enormous conflicts arise when one adult feels another is not feeding her child right. Fasting is a potential source of conflict. If a parent believes that fasting brings one closer to God and thus is trying to elevate their child's spirituality, they'll be shocked if the child care center reports them for neglect. If the adults don't learn to manage this conflict (if they can't resolve it), a difficult situation will exist. If the teacher or caregiver regards the parent as bad because he or she feels the child is being deprived, strong feelings can arise that create unfortunate behaviors, such as feeding a fasting child or giving meat to a vegetarian. The conflict is especially painful if the teacher or caregiver has to deal with a child crying when the other children are being served.

Taking Responsibility for the Amount that a Child Eats

Another potential area of conflict arises around taking or not taking responsibility for how much children eat. Parenting experts oppose urging or forcing children to eat, citing *body wisdom* as the reason. Babies will eat when they are hungry because of the body's natural inclination to keep itself healthy. Babies have a way of getting what they need when offered a balanced diet, agree the experts. All advise not to force, coax, or bribe. Those behaviors on the part of parents, teachers and caregivers lead to eating problems in children.[7]

Only in families where there is an abundance of food is getting children to eat an issue. On a worldwide basis, urging or forcing children to eat is seldom thought about. According to Werner:

> Three-quarters of all the world's children under the age of 15...live in developing countries. Every 30 seconds, 100 children are born somewhere in Asia, Africa, Latin America, or Oceania. Twenty of them will die within the year. Of the 80 who survive, 60 will suffer from malnutrition during the crucial weaning and toddler stage, with the possibility of irreversible stunting of physical and mental growth.[8]

The parents of these children don't face the problem of urging their children to eat—their worry is getting the food to offer them. Starving children need no urging.

Parents who have access to adequate amounts of food but have witnessed the starvation of others often feel it is their job to get a certain amount of food into their children. Many cultures value chubby children, perhaps because thin children tend to die. But beyond that factor, many cultures see chubby as attractive and desirable. According to Stringfellow, Liem, and Liem, of forty-one Vietnamese parents asked, all said they thought that babies should be fat.[9]

Parents who manage to keep their children the size most admired feel they are doing a good job as parents. Parents of thin children may feel inadequate. Thinness, instead of being looked upon as healthy, as it is to some extent in the mainstream culture, may be regarded as a sign of weak health in other cultures.

Sometimes the parent sees the teacher's or caregiver's job as making sure the child eats the "right amount," which is fine as long as that expectation corresponds with the child's appetite. However, when the "right amount" is either more or less than the child wants to eat, and the caregiver feels the child's natural body wisdom should determine the amount consumed, a conflict is in the making. It is hard to convince most caregivers who have the "when you're done, you're done" attitude to work at getting extra food into a child. It's also hard for caregivers to cut off the food supplies when a child is still hungry unless they see a strong reason for doing so.

Using Food to Pacify

Feeding as a response to unhappiness is another common area of conflict between caregivers and parents. Some babies will settle down with a bottle whether or not they are hungry. Often caregivers feel strongly that babies should not be pacified with food because it sets up a lifelong tendency to look to food for comfort.

They may also feel that it is all right for babies to cry when they are express-ing discomfort, dissatisfaction, or anger. If a parent who is used to pacifying with a bottle walks in and sees his or her child crying her eyes out, the parent will probably be unhappy with the caregiver. This issue goes beyond food and includes whether or not a child should be allowed or encouraged to express feel-ings, even angry and unhappy ones. This issue is discussed in Chapter Seven.

In conclusion, some of these cultural differences in feeding practices reflect conflicting values. If the child is to grow up to be self-sufficient, independent, competitive, assertive—a unique individual—it's possible that parents will value feeding practices that stress early self-help skills and competence building. Ironically, however, holding infants when they drink from a bottle is often valued because it is considered a step toward independence. A connection is made between fulfilling attachment needs and later independence. Secure, attached children—those who are held when fed—it is believed, grow up to be more inde-pendent than those left to fend for themselves alone in a crib with a propped bottle.

In families where the goal is for the child to remain close to the family, not to grow up to be an independent person living apart and perhaps alone, the stress is on interdependence. Caregiving practices, including feeding routines, reflect the fact that parents do not stress individuality and independence but rather cooperation and connectedness, both in the present and as a future goal.

SUMMARY OF SUGGESTIONS FOR RESOLVING CONFLICTS OVER EATING AND SLEEPING

Here are some steps you can take when you find yourself on the opposite side from a parent in a conflict over sleeping or feeding issues:

1. Sort out whether this is an important issue or not. Is the parent's prac-tice actually harming the child? The issue may concern whether to hold the babies to put them to sleep or to let them sleep with their parents. This issue may not be important. Talk with others as part of this sorting process. Upon close examination, you may see that there is no potential harm and that it is just a difference of opinion. Neither of you is right or wrong. If this is the case, perhaps you can let go of the issue. What about the situation of a baby sleeping with a bottle? What about the risks of "bottle mouth?" (Bottle mouth is a term for tooth decay caused by for-mula, milk, or juice bathing the teeth for long hours during sleep.) In addition, as mentioned in Chapter One, there's an issue regarding the risks of putting young babies to sleep on their stomachs. If you know that the baby has a higher chance of dying of Sudden Infant Death

Syndrome (SIDS), could you just go along with what the parent says if he says place the baby in a prone position?

2. If you can't let go of it, try looking at the issue from the parent's perspective. This may not be easy if you don't have experience with changing perspectives. But if you work with young children, you probably have had experience at seeing the world through a child's eyes. Try now seeing this situation through a particular adult's eyes. An important prerequisite for seeing a new view is not to get angry or defensive. That's easier said than done if this conflict has triggered strong feelings in you. See if you can set aside those feelings and ask yourself, "Do I understand this parent's goals for his child?"

3. Help the parent articulate his or her goals. This probably won't happen overnight. It is most likely to happen as the result of a rather lengthy, ongoing dialogue. Once you both understand what the parent wants for his or her child, you can together examine whether or not the practice in question reflects those goals. If the practice and the goals fit, you should reconsider your own position in the matter. However, if the practice and goals conflict, you have your job cut out for you.

4. The ideal situation is when, with or without your efforts, parents come to see on their own that the practice and the goals are in conflict and figure out what to do about that situation. They may want your advice at this point if you haven't been too pushy about your own point of view from the start. Now the parents may decide to change the practice to be more in accordance with personal or cultural goals.

FOR FURTHER READING

Chang, Hedy. *Affirming Children's Roots: Cultural and Linguistic Diversity in Early Care and Education.* San Francisco: California Tomorrow, 1993. Examines, among other things, cultural deficiencies in programs, some of which focus on caregiving routines.

Clark, A. L., ed. *Culture and Childrearing.* Philadelphia: F. A. Davis, 1981. Gives a good overview of child-rearing practices as described by members of various cultures.

Gonzalez-Mena, Janet. *A Caregiver's Guide to Routines in Infant-Toddler Care.* Sacramento: Child Development Division, Center for Child and Family Studies, Far West Laboratory for Educational Research and Development, California Department of Education, 1990. Discusses eating and sleeping routines in infant-toddler programs.

Gonzalez-Mena, Janet, "Cultural Sensitivity in Routine Caregiving Tasks," in Mangione, Peter, ed., *Infant/Toddler Caregiving: A Guide to Culturally Sensitive Care.* Sacramento, Calif.: Far West Laboratory and California Department of Education, 1995. Looks at cross-cultural issues in feeding and other caregiving routines.

Morelli, G., Rogoff, B., and Oppenheim, D., "Cultural Variation in Infants' Sleeping Arrangements: Questions of Independence," *Developmental Psychology*, 28(4). Examines sleeping as it relates to independence.

Phillips, Carol Brunson, and Cooper, Renatta M., "Cultural Dimensions of Feeding Relationships," *Zero to Three* 12(5), June 1992, 10-13. More about culture and infant feeding.

NOTES

1.   Dorothy Lee describes the pattern one person, going beyond the issue of separate sleeping arrangements to the larger issue of separation. She says not only do babies sleep separately in cribs, but individuals are kept apart in many other ways even when they are mothers and babies. "In our society, clothing separates mother and child; is it to protect each from the hazards of a sudden draft? It was 102°F in my hospital room when I was first allowed to hold my baby; yet both baby and mother were carefully swathed in cloth which kept them to that degree distinct. Clothing, in fact, guards everyone against cutaneous contact with others, except perhaps, at the beach. We have divided our benches into individual units, our seats in school, on the train, on the bus. Even our solid sofas, planned for social grouping, have demarcating lines or separate pillows to help individuals keep apart." Obviously, a separate crib makes sense to a culture where individuals are kept apart from each other. Lee, Dorothy, *Freedom and Culture*. Englewood Cliffs, N.J.: Prentice-Hall, 1959, p. 31.

2.   The following references describe pattern two cultures. Young writes of African-American families: "In many cases, the physical closeness between infants and adults is reinforced by the fact that they are often observed to sleep with their parents or either parent alone. There is a kind of rhythm found between eating and napping with short periods of each activity found with frequent repetition. This rhythm is very different from the disciplined long span of attention cultivated in middle-class child-rearing and expected in schools. Virginia Young, 1970, quoted in Hale-Benson, Janice E., *Black Children: Their Roots, Culture, and Learning Styles*. Baltimore: Johns Hopkins University Press, 1986, p. 70.

Morrow says that Vietnamese, Cambodian, and Laotian children often sleep with their parents, Cambodian children sometimes up to ten years of age. Morrow, Robert D., "Cultural Differences—Be Aware!" *Academic Therapy* 23(2), November 1987, p. 147.

Caudill and Plath looked at sleeping arrangements in Japanese families. They found that the father and mother often slept in separate rooms, each with a child or children. The grandmother was also likely to sleep with a child. Caudill, W., and Plath, D., "Who Sleeps by Whom? Parent-Child Involvement in Urban Japanese Families," *Psychiatry* 29(4), 1966, 344–366.

According to Werner, "in a great majority of societies infants sleep in the same bed with their mothers during the time they are nursing—the first 2 to 3 years. In less than 10 of the world's societies whose ethnographies were surveyed did infants sleep in a crib or cradle of their own. Even where infants have a cradle or cot of their own, it is generally placed near the mother's bed within easy reach. Only in Western societies, notably middle-class United States, do infants have a bedroom of their own. In slightly less than one-half of the societies under consideration, the father also shared the bed with mother and infant. In slightly over half of the societies of the world, the husband slept in a bed in the same room but at some distance from his wife, or in another room." Werner, E., *Cross-Cultural Child Development: A View from the Planet Earth*. Monterey, Calif.: Brooks/Cole, 1979, p. 270.

In describing a pattern two culture, the Tikopia, Lee discusses sleeping arrangements and their relationship to individuals: "the Tikopia help the self to be continuous with its society through their physical arrangements. They find it good to sleep side by side crowding each other, next to their children or their parents or their brothers and sisters, mixing sexes and generations." Lee, *Freedom and Culture*, p. 31.

3. According to Shinnamon, "Hand feeding of children, sometimes through age four, is fairly common throughout the world. When this practice is analyzed objectively we can see that it is a logical adaptation that mothers and caretakers make in environments where 1) mothers are essential workers in the economy and have a short amount of time each day to devote to children's feeding; 2) water, which is necessary for washing baby's hands, face and clothes, may be scarce; 3) food is in short supply and cannot be wasted by allowing a baby or young child to feed itself...the ability to allow a baby freedom to feed itself, with all the mess and waste that goes with it, is a definite luxury which few people in the world can afford." Shinnamon, Felicia, "Childhood: A Multicultural Perspective," unpublished manuscript, p. 6.

4. Comer, J. P., and Poussaint, A. F., *Black Child Care*. New York: Simon and Schuster, 1975.

5. Leach, P., *Your Baby and Child from Birth to Age Five*. New York: Alfred A. Knopf, 1987. Spock, B., and Rothenberg, M., *Dr. Spock's Baby and Child Care*. New York: E. P. Dutton, 1985.

6. Sodetaini-Shibata, Aimee Emiko, "The Japanese American," in *Culture and Childrearing*, A. L. Clark, ed. Philadelphia: F. A. Davis, 1981, p. 98.

7. Beebe, B. M., *Best Bets for Babies*. New York: Dell, 1981. See also Comer and Poussaint, *Black Child Care*, Leach; *Your Baby and Child*; and Spock and Rothenberg, *Dr. Spock's Baby*.

8. Werner, *Cross-Cultural Child Development*, p. 1.

9. Stringfellow, L., Liem, N. D., and Liem, L., "The Vietnamese in America," in *Culture and Childrearing*, Ann L. Clark, ed. Philadelphia: F. A. Davis, 1981, p. 235.

CHAPTER FIVE

Attachment and Separation

Compare these two three month old babies at home with their mothers.

BABY A

Baby A is on her back on a blanket in the middle of the floor. Her mother, also on the floor, sits in front of her and is leaning over looking into her eyes. They are playing a little game. Baby goes "agggg" and laughs. Mother imitates her. Baby repeats the sound. Then her mother goes "agggg" and clicks her tongue three times. Baby imitates her sound exactly, waving her arms toward her mother's face. The only sound in the house is of the two voices.

The phone rings, shattering the stillness and interrupting their play. The mother says to her baby, "There's the phone. I have to go answer it. I'll be right back." She gets up as she speaks, picking up a toy as she does so. She shakes the toy, which has a bell in it, and when the baby's eyes grasp the toy, she sets it down by the baby's face within easy reach. She moves quickly away and out the door. The baby's face clouds up as she watches her mother's retreating back. When she disappears, the baby lets out a loud howl. "Yes, yes, I know you don't want me to leave. I'm right here in the other room. I'll be back." The sound of her mother's voice temporarily reassures the baby, and she turns her attention to the toy by her ear.

If we follow this mother around for a whole Saturday (she works during the week), we find that she and her baby spend periods together and periods apart.

The mother values "time to herself" and feels the baby needs privacy and "alone time" as well, so she arranges the day that way.

Here are the ways the baby gets "alone time": she sleeps in her crib in her room during her two naps; she spends time by herself on the floor and is sometimes in a playpen while her mother is occupied elsewhere in the house.

She's also away from her parents periodically in the evening. They get a babysitter and go out fairly often—because they need "couple time."

Although Baby A is apart from her mother regularly, when they are together, her mother often gives her full attention to her daughter, as in the previous scene. She talks to her, plays little games with her, shows her toys, and responds to what the baby initiates. She spends "quality time" with her.

This mother thinks about attachment. She's aware of the term and of its importance. She knows that attachment comes from being sensitive to her daughter. She understands the importance of interactions in promoting attachment. She knows that she is her daughter's primary attachment. The baby's father is also part of the picture, and the baby is attached to him, too, but prefers her mother when both parents are together.

The mother feels confident that putting her daughter into child care has not hurt their attachment. She knows that her daughter recognizes her and has noticed that she responds to her differently than she responds to the caregivers in the program. Once in a while she worries that her daughter will become too attached to one of the caregivers, but then she recognizes that this is just normal jealousy on her part—mothers are supposed to be possessive. She is able to reassure herself that in the long run, she's the one who really counts.

BABY B

Now look at Baby B. She is on her grandmother's lap, sitting up, looking outward. She slumps over and contentedly sucks and nibbles on her grandmother's arm, glancing up occasionally to look at the people in the room. Her grandmother is having a conversation with her mother, who is sitting on the other end of the couch. The baby's aunt is sewing in one corner of the room, and two cousins are watching TV in another corner. Now and then the baby makes a fussing sound, and the grandmother jiggles her or strokes her back without taking her attention away from the conversation she's deeply engrossed in.

The TV watchers leave the room, and the grandmother gets up and turns down the volume, taking the baby with her on her arm. As the grandmother walks back toward her seat, the baby's mother holds out her arms, and the grandmother deposits the baby in her lap. The children come back in and turn up the volume of the TV again. The mother rocks the baby, matching the rhythm of a commercial issuing from the TV.

The phone rings. The mother gets up and answers it. She holds the baby while she's talking on the phone, but when the baby starts to fuss, the aunt gets up from her sewing machine and comes to take the baby out of her arms, walking her around the room, bouncing her gently.

The baby quickly falls asleep in her aunt's arms. The woman carefully puts her down on the couch beside the grandmother. She goes back to her sewing machine and in a few minutes announces to one of the TV watchers, "Well, your dress is done—just in time for the party tonight. Go try it on." That rouses the rest of the group, who get up and leave the room, presumably to start getting ready. Only the grandmother is left in the room, sitting by the baby on the couch until the mother comes to relieve her. The mother arrives from the other room, bringing the special outfit she plans for the baby to wear to the party.

This baby is never alone. She is always in someone's arms or near them. When the family goes somewhere, she goes too, like to the party they're all getting ready for.

The family thinks very little about this baby's attachment. There's always been a baby or two in the house and always plenty of people to take care of them. The concept of infant attachment isn't something this family worries about.

This baby has multiple caregivers, and the mother sees it as an asset, wondering what she'd ever do if she were the only one responsible for her baby. She shudders at the thought.

In this family, the attachment issues (though they don't call them that) lie beyond infancy. The concern of the older family members is not about whether the babies are attached or not, but how to keep the generation that has just reached adulthood tied to the family when so many forces pull it away. It's a special worry for the grandmother, who has one son in college in another city. Will he come back when he becomes a lawyer? And her youngest daughter recently married a man who is in the service. So far she is still at home, but when her husband is stationed someplace where she can join him, what will happen?

A THEME IN ATTACHMENT: CUTTING OR NOT CUTTING THE APRON STRINGS

Edward T. Hall, in his book *Beyond Culture*, says: "The world is divided into those cultures who cut the apron strings and those who do not."[1]

Baby B lives in a family where growing up has not traditionally been a matter of cutting apron strings. The adults in the family in the past have not had to establish their own identity independent of their parents. They became mature adults while remaining part of their extended family. They didn't consider alternatives.[2]

According to Francis Hsu, in his culture, "the parent-child ties are permanent rather than transitory. It is taken for granted that they are immutable, and so are not subject to individual acceptance or rejection."[3]

Baby A's mother is from a culture that cuts the apron strings. Ironically, her concern is about tying her baby to the apron strings in the first place. Because her child is in care outside the home, attachment is an issue for her. But she has also begun the process of making her baby into a separate individual in anticipation of cutting the strings eventually. For her, the two processes of attachment and separation are an intertwining theme to be played out together throughout the child's life. She expects someday her daughter will move away from home, from parents, and make her own life elsewhere, just as she did.

Baby A, in contrast to Baby B, is being encouraged to attach to one person—her mother. Although she has secondary attachments—her father and perhaps a caregiver at the program where she goes—her mother is the most important person in her life. Their interactions, especially when coupled with caregiving routines such as feeding, tend to produce the kind of infant attachment valued by Baby A's mother's culture. She is already showing differentiated reactions—demonstrating her attachment to her mother. In a few more months, she may also begin to show fear of people she doesn't know and may begin to protest mightily at being separated from her mother. Many children with this kind of attachment begin to exhibit what is called "separation anxiety" at about nine months of age, crying when the parent leaves even though they have been in day care for some time and never protested before.

Baby B is used to multiple caregivers, which brings various personalities into her life. She probably won't experience the pulls of the exclusive relationship that Baby A has or the feelings of jealousy among the adults in her life.[4] Both Baby B and Baby A are too young to show separation anxiety. But because Baby B is always with at least one of her caregivers, she probably won't show it when she is older either. However, if she were to be left with a stranger, she'd probably protest even louder than Baby A and at an earlier age as well.[5] Some babies with a strong group connection get very upset when away from the group they identify with.

Baby A and Baby B illustrate a set of priorities rather than two absolutes. Although the goal of Baby A's parents is to produce an individual who can stand on her own feet by herself, they aren't excluding the social needs of their daughter. Of course they want her to feel close to people and to get along with them. They want her to be able to commit to relationships, both inside and outside the family. They don't intend that their daughter will eventually move away and shun her parents. And, of course, Baby B's family wants her to be able to function in the world beyond the family, to attain a measure of individuality.

It's the degree of separateness that makes the difference in the goals for Baby A and Baby B. It's also the fact that Baby A's parents expect their daughter to be able to move in and out of relationships and be able to break off any relationship that takes away her freedom to be an individual. Baby B's family doesn't have this same goal of breaking off relationships when they begin to pinch. They expect their daughter to work out things *within* the relationship, not leave it behind and move on.

THE INFLUENCE OF LIFE THREATS ON THE ATTACHMENT PROCESS

Life-threatening situations may influence the nature of early attachment. A premature baby or a very sick one may not have the kind of behaviors that promote attachment, automatically endearing parents and others to him or her. Some adults become attached in spite of the baby's lack of ability to promote the attachment. However, in other cases, family members distance themselves either consciously or unconsciously because they fear the pain of the potential loss.

It's not that preemies or sick newborns never develop attachment; it's just that the patterns can differ from those of healthy newborns. This may not be a permanent disruption. The attachment may well occur when the crisis is past or later even with the life-threatening situation still present.

This relates to my experience of life-threatening situations as they occur among middle-class Americans. It's not a major theme of most U.S. families; it's an individual situation—isolated incidents. However, some families around the world experience infant death as a theme in their lives. I'm not talking about long, long ago; high mortality rates in the first five years are still the norm worldwide.[6] They are also higher than you might expect in some areas of the United States.

When I first started working in an early childhood program, I worked with low-income Mexican immigrant parents and their children. I remember, now and then, asking the parents how how many brothers and sisters they had. Each gave me two answers—the number born and the number left alive. That was a different experience for me because until then, I didn't know anyone in my generation who had lost brothers or sisters.

If you've always lived in a population where infant survival seems assured, you may have a hard time understanding the possible effect of a high infant mortality rate on child-rearing practices. Imagine what it must be like to live in a family where babies have died—not only recently, but for generations. Experiences with the constant threat of infant death influence the way parents behave.

Parent Behaviors

Parents in these circumstances or with this background concentrate on ways to save the baby rather than on ways to develop physical or intellectual skills, as do parents who have little or no experience of infant mortality. But "saving the baby" is so ingrained into the child-rearing practices that it isn't thought of in those terms. Those in this situation would probably not explain to you in those particular terms why they are doing what they do. They accept what they are doing as normal child-rearing practices. It's what they're used to, what they were raised with. Outsiders call them cultural practices.

Here are some common patterns of infant care in Africa, Latin America, and Indonesia in populations with high infant mortality rates:

1. The infant is on or near a caretaker's body at all times, day and night.
2. Crying is quickly attended to and becomes rare relative to Western infants.
3. Feeding is a very frequent response to crying.
4. There is, by Western standards, little organized concern about the infants' behavioral development and relatively little treatment of them as emotionally responsive individuals (as in eye contact, smile elicitation, or chatting).[7]

What do these characteristics have to do with promoting survival? LeVine says:

> The infant is kept on or near a caretaker at all times so his condition can be monitored. His cries are immediately attended to so that the caretaker can receive immediate feedback concerning whether they are easily reduced by shaking or feeding; if not, perhaps he is ill. Minimizing his crying from other causes heightens the value of crying as a signal of organic upset, i.e., disease. Frequent feeding, particularly breast-feeding, serves to replace fluids and alleviate the dehydration from diarrhea that is probably the most frequent precipitant of infant death in the tropics. Keeping the infant on someone's body or otherwise restricted prevents the accidental injuries that can lead to death if not properly treated. All in all, though not a highly effective medical system, it is an adaptive response to extreme environmental hazard and probably has more efficacy than is readily apparent....In this pattern of infant care adapted to the risks of disease and death in the earliest years, there is no place for an organized concern about the development of the child's behavioral characteristics and social and emotional relationships; such concerns are postponed until later in his life, when custom provides a basis for confidence in his continued survival.[8]

Separating Survival Practices from Cultural Values

Now the question is what happens to the infant care practices after the circumstances change. Suppose the family moves to this country, finds relative economic security and good medical care, and the risks to their babies drop drastically. Maybe no baby dies in this family for several generations. Do the infant care practices change?

LeVine's theory is that they continue on after the threat is passed, perhaps for generations. These customs become ingrained in the cultural approach to infant care. My theory is that it is hard to separate these survival practices from cultural values and attachment patterns.

The issue is whether you have to. If you're in the position of doing parent education or find yourself working with a child for whom you have some concerns, you're going to have a dilemma about what to do with a family, for example, that doesn't seem sensitive to the baby's emotional signals, seldom speaks to their baby, or never holds the baby in a face-to-face position so adult and baby can make eye contact. What if the baby is never called by name but rather by a variety of nicknames, some of which may be derogatory, or even called nothing at all? How do these behavior patterns fit into the family's cultural values? Are they leftover survival practices, or do they relate to the family's goals for their baby? What about language? Will the baby learn by just hearing language but not being spoken to? Is the family using nonverbal communication that the outsider isn't aware of, or is there a lack of communication? Is there an attachment problem or just a cultural difference?

These are not easy questions, and your answers will depend on how well you, while being supersensitive to cultural differences, judge how well the behaviors are serving the child and the family. Of course, you don't have to judge unless you're in a position that makes you an interventionist. Then you have to ask whether intervening with this family is appropriate or not. This kind of judgment is best made by a skilled and trained person of the same culture as the family, but that's not always possible.

Here's an example of a cultural practice that was complicated by other factors. The issue was infant mobility. The setting was a day-care center for migrant farm workers. The director of the program, who was of the same culture as the parents, insisted that babies be given freedom to move around by being put on the floor. She felt that holding the babies all the time or keeping them restricted in other ways shortchanged their development. The parents protested that it wasn't their way. Babies shouldn't be on the floor. And indeed, in their homes, the floor was dangerous. With a number of people who work outdoors living in a small space, there was no telling what might be on the floor in addition to dirt (no matter how often it was swept) and possibly splinters. Besides, you don't leave babies to be stepped on in small, crowded rooms.[9] Being on the floor in the clean, spacious center was very different from being on the floor at home; yet the parents still resisted the idea.

The director understood the parents' perspective, why they held their babies all the time and why, in the center, they expected someone to hold their babies or at least keep them in cribs or infant swings. She wanted to respect the parents' wishes, but at the same time, she had seen with her own eyes the way unrestricted infants develop, moving their bodies freely. She wanted the best for the babies in her center, and she knew the parents did too. They just didn't know any way other than the one they were used to. The director- was finally able to convince the parents that she wasn't taking the children's culture from them by carrying out a practice different from what they were used to at home.

Another example of a practice that may seem culturally related but is more related to survival issues is that of not calling a baby by name. This practice is a self-protection measure that may follow the previous loss of a child. I personally understand this because I had a premature baby who was in intensive care for three months. I tried to protect myself because I thought I might lose my son at any time. I even called him by a name different than the one on his birth certificate. After experiencing this situation, I became very sensitive to the concerns of parents. I never try to "educate" parents by telling them that it is important to use the baby's name. I remember one child in the intensive care nursery who never even received a name from her parents. She wasn't visited very often, either. It's easy to criticize other parents until you experience the prospect of losing a baby. Every instinct tells you not to get attached to the baby. For me, I'm pleased to report that attachment came later—a strong, healthy attachment. I don't know about the nameless baby. Once she left the intensive care nursery, I never saw or heard anything about her again.[10]

CONCLUSION

The attachment patterns illustrated in the first part of this chapter show the difference between independence and interdependence as goals. Baby A is being trained in an independence mode; Baby B's family values interdependence. Both goals aim at producing fully functioning, competent individuals. The difference between the two patterns is in the outcome. Baby B's family values lifelong attachment to the group; Baby A's family aims to produce a separate and unique individual who can stand alone. But the comparison demands highlighting the differences—looking at extremes. In reality, it's a matter of balance. Baby A's family wants her to relate to the group, gain social competencies. They emphasize the individuality within a group context. Baby B's family needs a fully functioning individual who knows who she is and what she can do. They focus on her embeddedness rather than on her individuality.

How do you differentiate between cultural differences and dysfunction—especially in the area of attachment? It's not easy unless you are able to look at a family through its cultural eyes. This important question has no easy answer. If you're not careful, you may look at a dysfunctional family in a culture different from yours and decide its behaviors are cultural, without seeing how they hurt the members of that family. It's also possible to look at a functional family through your own cultural eyes and decide that, because it's different, it's dys-

functional. That's why we need more education and experience when we cross
cultures than when we work in a monocultural setting.

FOR FURTHER READING

Bowlby, J. *Attachment and Loss: Vol. 1: Attachment.* New York: Basic Books, 1969. A classic book on attachment theory.

Hall, Edward T., *Beyond Culture.* Garden City, New York: Anchor Books, 1977. No specific discussion about attachment, but it does mention attachment among other subjects.

Levine, Robert A., "A Cross-Cultural Perspective on Parenting," in Fantini, M. D. and Cardenas, R. (eds.), *Parenting in a Multicultural Society.* New York: Longman, 1980, 17–26. A cross-cultural view of parenting issues, including attachment.

Levine, Robert A., "Child Rearing as Cultural Adaptation" in Leiderman, P. Herbert, Tulkin, Steven R. and Rosenfeld, Anne (eds.), *Culture and Infancy: Variations in the Human Experience.* New York and San Francisco: Academic Press, 1977. Attachment may be influenced by survival issues.

Lubeck, Sally, *The Sandbox Society: Early Education in Black and White America.* Philadelphia: The Falmer Press, 1985. An interesting look at cultural differences in preschool including a comparison between collective and individualistic orientation.

NOTES

1. Hall, Edward T., *Beyond Culture.* Garden City, N.Y.: Anchor Press/Doubleday, 1981, .p. 226. Hall also says, "In many cultures, the bonds with the parents, grandparents, and even ancestors are not severed but are maintained and reinforced. I am thinking of China, Japan, the traditional Jewish family of central Europe, the Arab villagers, the Spanish of North and South America, and the Pueblo Indians of New Mexico, to mention only a few." Children move from childhood to adulthood, but they do not establish lives of their own, identities separate from their parents—their people.

2. Other writers and researchers discuss this view of lifelong attachment found in Baby B's family. Dorothy Lee says of the Hopi: "Loyalties are to the group; they are not person-to-person loyalties. And parents have been known deliberately to try to shift a child's affection from concentration upon one family member, to diffusion among the group." Lee, Dorothy, *Freedom and Culture.* Englewood Cliffs, N.J.: Prentice-Hall, 1959, p. 20.

    Sally Lubeck says of African-American families: "From an early age, a Black child is likely to live in an extended family, with grandparents, aunts, uncles or cousins, as well as siblings, likely, as people move in and out with changing circumstances, to have a broadened sense of 'family.' A Black child is far more likely to sleep with others, to experience less privacy (and also less loneliness) than a White American child.

A child will frequently be nurtured and supervised by more than one primary adult." Lubeck, Sally, *Sandbox Society: Early Education in Black and White America*. Philadelphia: Falmer Press, 1985, p. 110.

Lubeck also talks of two patterns, which she calls a collective orientation versus an individualistic orientation. "A collective orientation is apparent when enculturation occurs in a shared function environment where the focus is on social relations, stressing 'kinship,' interdependency, and cooperation, a holistic world view, relational thinking, and the importance of non-verbal communication. An individualistic orientation predominates when enculturation occurs in a nucleated family structure, focusing on manipulator experience and stressing self-achievement, competition, the ability to abstract parts from wholes, abstract thinking and the importance of verbal communication." Lubeck, *Sandbox Society*, p. 40.

Matthiessen says of the Hmong: "Hmong households are usually composed of several generations, including married sons and their families. It is expected that children, especially the youngest of the family, will care for their parents as they grow old." Matthiessen, Neba, *The Hmong: A Multicultural Study*. Fairfield, Calif.: Fairfield-Suisun Unified School District, 1987, p. 7.

Trinh Ngoc Dung says of the Vietnamese: "Traditionally, a Vietnamese family may consist of three or perhaps four generations. Daughters, when married, join their husbands' families." Trinh Ngoc Dung, "Understanding Asian Families: A Vietnamese Perspective," *Children Today*, March–April 1984, p. 11.

Duong Thanh Binh says of the Vietnamese: "The majority of Vietnamese are deeply attached to their families. Feelings of family honor, duty, and responsibility are very strong, even in the very young." Duong Thanh Binh, *A Handbook for Teachers of Vietnamese Students: Hints for Dealing with Cultural Differences in Schools*. Arlington, Vir.: Center for Applied Linguistics, 1975, p. 13.

3. Hsu, Francis L. K., *Americans and Chinese: Purpose and Fulfillment in Great Civilizations*. Garden City, N.Y.: Natural History Press, 1970, p. 110.

4. Werner writes of families where "the responsibility for child care is shared among members of a homogeneous family group. Although the child may have a number of caretakers, they will all have a common set of socialization goals and a common set of practices in relation to child rearing. Child rearing is thus a collective rather than an individual responsibility....[T]he more people...there are in the house, the less exclusively attached to the mother is the infant. Intensity of affect, thus, may vary inversely with the number of caretakers, as Mead suggested...in her comparison of the Samoan extended family with the American nuclear family. Also fitting the Mead interpretation is the pattern reported for Israeli kibbutzim. In terms of the infant's development, several stable caretakers are seen as providing more stability than a single one, by lessening the stress of separation from the mother, for instance through the possibility of replacement by a second familiar caretaker." Werner, Emmy Elisabeth, *Cross-Culture Child Development*. Monterey, Calif.: Brooks/Cole, 1979, pp. 271, 275–276.

5. According to Mary Ainsworth, 1967, Ganda babies who grow up in an extended family exhibit separation protest as early as six months. Reported in Werner, *Cross-Culture Child Development*, p. 274.

6. According to Werner: "Three-quarters of all the world's children under the age of 15 ...live in the developing countries. Every 30 seconds, 100 children are born some-where in Asia, Africa, Latin America, or Oceania. Twenty of them will die within the year. Of the 80 who survive, 60 will have no access to modern medical care during their childhood. An equal number will suffer from malnutrition during the crucial weaning and toddler stage...during this period their chances of dying will be 20 to 40 times higher than if they lived in North America or Europe." Werner, *Cross-Culture Child Development*, p. 1.

    According to Garrett, the infant mortality rate was fifty percent for Hmong refugees in the jungle dependent on American supplies for survival. Garrett, W. E., "Thailand: Refuge from Terror," *National Geographic* 157, May 1980, p. 634. See also Garrett, W. E., "The Hmong of Laos: No Place to Run," *National Geographic* 145, January 1974, 78–111.

7. LeVine, Robert A., "Child Rearing as Cultural Adaptation," in *Culture and Infancy: Variations in the Human Experience*, P. Herbert Leiderman, Steven R. Tulkin, and Anne Rosenfeld, eds. New York: Academic Press, 1977, p. 23.

8. Ibid., p. 25.

9. Although the example given was not the Hmong culture, this is what Campbell says: "the average Hmong family consists of 6–8 members who live in small apartments." Campbell, Kate, "Energy Program Helps Refugees Make Transition to Life in the U.S.," *PG&E Progress*, April 1985, p. 6.

10. My son has never been called by the name we chose for him before his birth. Without realizing it, we followed a family tradition regarding names. My father-in-law was the third boy born to his parents. The other two died in infancy. The first two were named after their father, Francisco. When the third boy, my father-in-law, was born, his parents named him Sergio. At age two, my father-in-law's parents changed his name from Sergio to Francisco. Perhaps they thought they had outwitted fate which seemed to kill all of their babies named Francisco. I don't know. I just know that my father-in-law and my son were named one name but called another, and that issues of survival were involved in this name change.

CHAPTER SIX

Play and Exploration

W hat this chapter is really about is learning. Children, from infancy on, learn through everything that happens to them (as well as the things they cause to happen). They learn as teachers and caregivers interact with them during caregiving times and daily routines and even when they don't interact with them. They learn when they play. ✓

How an adult regards play, facilitates it, plans for it, sets up the environment, and interacts with the child are all influenced by that adult's culture. Play may be valued or not. Culture helps determine whether play is seen as something that children do on their own with no adult involvement or whether adult involvement is valuable. Culture also may determine whether children spend most of their time in a child-centered environment—one set up for them with child size furniture, equipment, and toys. Some adults prefer children to be in an adult centered environment.

Even when two adults agree that young children should spend at least some of their time in a child-centered environment, they may differ about how the children should use this environment. One may see play as an opportunity for individual involvement with the physical environment, as in self-motivated, solitary play. Another adult may regard play as an opportunity for learning to get along with others. If solitary play is valued, interruptions by others will be discouraged (like the kind of protection for the individual provided in some Montessori programs). If play is regarded primarily as socialization, the adult will encourage children to interact. Imagine infants and toddlers playing and learning.

Two eighteen month olds are rolling around and tussling over a partially deflated beach ball. Their squeals of laughter are the main sounds heard in the room containing two caregivers and eight children from six months to twenty months of age. These two frolickers continually bump up against a low, carpet-covered divider that is part of an enclosure containing a six month old and a seven month old who are lying side by side on a rug looking at each other through a forest of toys. The two gurgle and coo periodically, their voices intermingling with the squeals coming from the other side of the divider.

A fourteen month old toddles over to the divider. She is pushing a toy on a stick. She abandons her stick and climbs over the divider, plops herself down between the two babies, and touches the younger one gently on the face. An adult immediately appears and sits down with the three children inside the enclosure. She doesn't do anything but says, "You like to touch Ana's face." It is obvious that she is ready to protect the immobile child if the need arises. The girl starts playing with the toys scattered around the floor, and the baby starts to fuss with the attention gone. The girl gets up and leaves, and the caregiver says, "You liked her to play with you." Then she hands the baby a plastic toy, which she waves and bangs contentedly. The caregiver turns to the seven month old, who has been rolling back and forth, pulling at her, and producing a series of sounds accompanied by bubbles. The two begin a "conversation." The caregiver imitates the baby at first, then turns her own sounds into words, saying things like, "That's a funny noise you're making," "Oh look at your bubbles," and "I see what you're doing with your fingers!" She's teaching what is called "turn taking"—waiting each time for a response from the child before she takes the next turn at "conversation."

Across the room a fifteen month old climbs the stairs to a small slide and delights in going down head first, catching himself with his hands as he reaches the bottom. His laughter mingles with the squeals of the other two. He is watched by a nineteen month old who is tucked away in a small cubby under the slide.

The nineteen month old crawls out of the cubby and walks over to some two-piece puzzles laid out attractively on a very low wooden table. He picks up a piece in each hand and bangs them together. He turns to look at another child, who has pulled a hat down over his eyes and is prancing blindly up and down in front of a mirror giggling.

The room is quiet except for the periodic noises from the children. Even those are subdued because of the thick carpets, soft furniture, cloth wall hangings, and other sound absorbers.

The colors of the room are as subdued as the sounds. The walls and furnishings are natural tones—earthy, with just a touch of peach and quiet country blue accents here and there to liven them up. The toys, however, are bright primary colors, so they announce themselves, making splashes of color against the neutral background.

An adult is sitting quietly beside the child who is now trying on different hats from an array in a basket conveniently beside the mirror. The caregiver gets up unobtrusively and walks over to a record player. He announces to the child in the hat that he is going to play some "dancing" music. He puts on a classical piece, carefully adjusts the volume so the music is soft, and goes back to sit down by the child.

The two children with the beach ball have now begun to fight over it. The squeals are no longer happy as they tug and pull on the ball. The other caregiver comes over to the two and holds out a second ball. "Here, you can each have one," she says pleasantly. But they ignore her. One pulls harder and the ball comes out of the other's hands. He takes the ball and runs off to hide under the slide. The other follows and grabs the ball back; then the first child crawls out and slaps the child, who immediately looks for an adult to help. He's not disappointed. She's right there. She squats down between both boys, talking in soft, soothing tones. "Gently, gently," she demonstrates gentle touching. "Jason hurt you," she says to the boy who is now crying. She continues talking in an even, calm voice, describing what she thinks is going on within each child and discussing the interaction that just occurred. She doesn't criticize or judge. She just keeps talking in the same quiet vein. The crying stops. The energy gone from their conflict, both wander away, abandoning the caregiver and the beach ball.

"Snack time," announces the other caregiver cheerily, pointing to the clock and showing a tray of banana slices and raisins to the children. Several follow him to a little table. Others continue playing and ignore the interruption as if it never occurred.

ADULT REACTIONS TO THE AMOUNT OF STIMULATION IN THE SCENE

Here's how some adult observers reacted to this scene. "B-O-R-I-N-G!" says the first observer. "Not enough happening. It was so quiet and toned down I thought I'd go to sleep watching. If I was a baby there, I'd stir things up a bit," she says, winking. "And the music…" She wrinkles her nose in distaste. "It was much too quiet. Music with a good beat makes a place *alive*. I'd have the music going all the time, and I'd add some more activity and some color too!"

"I liked it," says another observer. "I thought it was just right. There was plenty happening. Any more and it would be chaos. If you have too much going on, children can't concentrate on any one thing. They lose their focus. The way this environment was set up was good; the quiet background allowed some aspects of the environment to claim the children's attention. For example, the muted colors let the toys be seen; and the muted sounds allowed the children to hear each other's voices clearly."

"I thought it was too noisy and busy," remarks still another observer. "I prefer a quieter setting for babies. All that wild screaming and laughing would disturb some children and stir others up to be wild themselves. The teachers should have tried to calm those wild kids down."

These are three different reactions to the amount of stimulation the scene provided. What one person feels is the optimum amount of sights, sounds, and movement, that is, sensory input, another feels bombards the children, and a third feels is boring. To some extent, this variation in sensory needs relates to individual preference and style, but it also connects to culture.

Some cultures wish to promote calm, placid styles of interaction and temperament, so they prefer less stimulating environments. They worry that the babies will get overstimulated in the exciting play and intense interactions if they aren't toned down. Some cultures value activity; others value stillness.[1] Active cultures promote exploration and movement for infants because these activities help develop problem-solving skills. However, there is another view. Meaningful inactivity is a concept that many adults have never heard of. Yet, in some cultures, being inactive is a valuable use of time. Dr. A. C. Ross (whose Lakota name is Ehanamani) points out that meditation can be a problem-solving method. Instead of actively engaging the environment or trying to reason out an answer through logic, one sits in silence. According to Ross's way of thinking, answers to problems come from the collective unconscious in moments of silence.

Other observers said, "I think there should be fewer toys. The children had too much to do—too many choices. The world isn't like that. Children need to learn to adapt and adjust to what's there, not be presented with a whole bunch of choices. We all need to learn to play the hand we're dealt, not act as if we could deal ourselves any hand we wanted."

"More teaching. Those caregivers weren't doing anything! I would have some learning objectives and have the adults work on them with the children."

"A fake world. Why put children in a place where the whole focus is them? I think children learn more when they tag along after adults who are doing real things in the real world. They can learn to help from an early age if they are part of adult life, not tucked away in a room where the adults are like robots just put there to serve them."

"More conversations. The adults were too quiet."

"Too much talking. The adult could have showed the kids how to handle the conflict rather than just talking about it. I thought she talked the thing to death!"

"It would be better if the adults talked to each other more—that's the way children learn: by being around adult conversations."

"Why didn't they hold the children? They all seemed so lonely to me."

"Why didn't they show the child how to work the puzzle—how to go down the slide properly?"

"I saw the caregiver look at her watch to see if it was snack time yet. Why not go by the children's hunger rather than the clock?"

"Why bring out another ball? I would have just put the one ball away when they started fighting over it."

"I like the way the environment is so efficiently set up that it frees the adult to be with the children during play times."

"I didn't like seeing those adults just sitting around doing nothing. I would have liked to see them cooking or cleaning or fixing broken toys or *something*. If they had more to do, the children would learn by watching adults do adult things."

"There was too much 'educational play.' I like watching children indulging in excesses. I love to stir them to hilarity, get them involved in nonsense. That's what they're supposed to do—run around knocking over blocks, yelling. That's what childhood is for! A good game of ring around the rosy sometimes will get them going."

These comments reflect a variety of value judgments about what's good for babies and toddlers in a play setting.

THEMES REFLECTED BY THE COMMENTS
People Versus Object Orientation

Standard early childhood practice emphasizes the importance of the physical environment. Anyone who is setting up an infant-toddler program will find lists and lists of toys and equipment readily available (often published by manufacturers). Books and articles have been written on how to arrange the environment so it is efficient for the adults, developmentally appropriate for the children, optimally challenging to encourage active exploration, and, above all, safe. If you ask the people who write these books and articles how important objects are for learning, you'd get a long, enthusiastic answer extolling the virtues of an abundance of developmentally appropriate *stuff* available for the children.

If you see the video of the research behind *Preschool in Three Cultures*, you'll be struck by the abundance of toys, materials, and equipment of the American program compared to both the Japanese and Chinese programs.[2] Depending on your point of view, you might say the Japanese and Chinese programs looked *stark*, or you might say the American program looked *stuffed*. No matter what your point of view, you're bound to notice the difference in the environments.

As a consumer society, we're surrounded with messages about the importance of owning *things*. When you combine those messages with a cultural value of objects, children receive a double dose of training toward object orientation. These messages affect the lives of even infants and toddlers.

Some cultures train their children to be more people oriented than object oriented. They put a focus on the social world rather than the physical world.

Young found that African-American families taught their children to pay more attention to person cues. They made it more important for them to focus on people than on objects by the way they interacted with their children. The style of interaction motivated the children to learn to judge the moods of people in authority. The interaction styles also included a great deal of touching, especially in the first three years of a child's life.[3]

When babies did focus on an object, picking up something on their own (it was not usually given to them), they were often redirected to the face of the person holding them. Because babies were held a lot, body contact figured prominently in child-rearing styles. Young believes that this approach to child rearing tends to move the child's interest away from the world of objects and redirects attention to people.

I was curious after reading Young to find out if people were aware that they trained their children to focus on the social world rather than on the world of objects, so I went around asking a number of people from a variety of cultures, both immigrants and native-born Americans, how important they thought it was for babies' development to have toys or objects to play with. Everyone I asked showed a strong leaning toward the importance of toys and other objects in the young child's environment. But what people say they believe is sometimes contradicted by their behavior. I think this attitude about toys for young children shows the selling job the early childhood people and the commercial world have done in getting people hooked on the idea that "educational toys" make a difference in cognitive development. I have noticed that some of these same people who claim the importance of toys still seem to emphasize people contact to their babies over pushing the toys they buy for "educational purposes."

Choice

Part of the reason for all these *things* in the environment in early childhood programs is that many people believe children need enough things to play with readily available so they can make choices. This emphasis on self-selection allows children to experience themselves as decision makers. It is based on a perception that individuals have power over their own lives and children need to learn to make choices from the beginning. It has to do with the goals of freedom of choice, self-direction, self-reliance, and independence. The point is to let children have the opportunity to choose from some number of options—the decisions about which options and how many lie in the hands of the adults. The theory is that children will learn to make the connections between their own choices and the consequences of those choices, so they will become skilled decision makers.

Not all adults are enthusiastic about giving children choices. They see a major task of childhood as learning to adapt to what is, to take advantage of what they find in the environment of adults, rather than selecting from a number of options that have been set up for them. They question the value of a child-oriented, developmentally appropriate environment isolated from the real world of adults. According to Jayanthi Mistry:

> In some cultural communities children learn by simply being present as adults go about their jobs and household activities. Adults do not create learning situations to teach their children. Rather, children have the responsibility to learn culturally valued behaviors and practices by observing and being around adults during the course of the day.[4]

There is a definite difference between setting up an environment specifically for children with scaled-down versions of adult implements and appliances (tea sets, miniature refrigerators, child-size carpentry sets, little garden tools, and such) and letting children be part of the adult environment to either observe or use real tools and appliances.

Hsu expands this view from the workaday world to the world of adult recreation and special occasions, saying, "Americans keep their children from the real world of adults—Chinese bring theirs with them to every occasion." He goes further to contrast the birthday parties that are centered on the birthday child, where the adults play the role of assistants or servants, which he has observed in America, to the child birthday parties that are adult occasions like wedding or funeral feasts. Anything that is child centered, in Hsu's opinion, isolates the child from "the real world of adults," which, in his mind, is a valuable environment for learning.[5]

Marta Borbon Ehling says something similar about Mexican-Americans: "Children usually go everywhere that their parents go. They go to parties, weddings, funerals, and church."[6]

Adult Role

The role of the adult is different in a child-centered environment than in an adult-centered environment. In the developmentally appropriate environment, the adult is often present as a facilitator of learning rather than as a teacher. After adults set up the environment, they back out of center stage. Their role is one of support as they encourage children's self-initiated explorations. They may also act as a resource, expanding on dramatic play, providing props and materials as needed. They refrain from taking over and directing the action. The idea is self-discovery. The adult may regularly add some questions or words to situations children choose, but straightforward teaching, either with words or through modeling, is usually not emphasized the way self-discovery is. Free play is free play, and the adult is more of a responder than anything else, leaving most goal-oriented inclinations out of his or her role. The role of adults in children's play, even in a child-centered environment, lies on a continuum. On one end, the adult is more observer than anything else; on the other end, the adult may be far more interactive with the children: entering the play, guiding, asking questions, making suggestions, and giving direction. In some programs, the adult takes ideas from the children's play and creates what Betty Jones and John Nimmo call an "emergent curriculum." In other words, some of the content in the plan for learning (including activities and projects) comes from the children rather than from an adult-centered curriculum.

This approach is in contrast to an adult role that emphasizes initiating, teaching, and directing. Some parents prefer that the teacher or caregiver remain in control of everything that happens. Parents understand schooling in terms of their own early experiences and are more comfortable with something familiar to them. A free-play situation in which adults take a more background role may be unsettling to parents. It may also be too child centered and appear too chaotic for some parents. What are the parent's feelings and ideas about these issues? Discuss them!

Your program doesn't have to be exactly what the parents feel is ideal for their children. It's okay for children to be exposed to environments and adult roles they aren't used to as long as parents don't believe that it's bad for their child and as long as children don't react adversely.

It's a give-and-take process. Mistry says, "When a caregiver respects and adapts to a child so too will that child become able to adapt to the caregiver and the child care setting created by that caregiver."[7] The same can be true of parents.

Children are good learners, and most are flexible enough to incorporate what you are adding to their lives. The important thing is if what you are doing is different from what they experience at home, it should be considered as an addition. **It's okay for children to become bicultural. It's not okay to take their home culture away from them.**

Emphasis on Words Versus Nonverbal Communication

Put two or more children together to play, and you'll have disputes. It's interesting to watch how adults handle conflicts between children. Some adults depend on words—on spelling things out, getting the cards on the table. Using a lot of words and expecting the children to learn to do that also is a characteristic of what is called a "low context culture."[8] Mainstream Canadian and U.S. cultures are low context cultures. High context cultures (like the Chinese culture) depend less on words than on other kinds of contextual messages. In some ways, two high context people communicate like two twins who know what the other means with minimal words.

This emphasizing or deemphasizing the verbal starts from the beginning with the way babies are treated. Babies carried around much of the time get good at sending messages nonverbally—through changing body position or tensing up or relaxing muscles, for example. They are encouraged to communicate this way when their caregivers pick up the messages they send. They don't need to depend on words at an early age. Babies who are physically apart from their caregivers learn the benefits of verbal communication. If the babies are on the floor in the infant program or in the other room at home, they need to learn to use their voices to get attention. Changing position or tensing muscles goes unperceived by the distant adult. (Babies at home also learn that silence will get them attention too, as a parent says, "Oh, oh, it's mighty quiet in there. I wonder what's going on!")

Adults who value verbal communication encourage babies to play with language. The "turn taking" in the previous scene is an example of an adult and child playing with language. Those who put a high value on verbal communication believe that babies learn through face-to-face "conversations," starting from birth on. This is a contrast to a different approach to language learning—that of "eavesdropping" (being around but not involved in adult conversations).[9]

Verbally oriented adults spend a lot of time paying attention to what children say and respond by clarifying and interpreting. They often expand on what the children are saying. They carry on conversations with them. While they are doing all this, they are modeling, without fanfare, correct speech.

Verbally oriented adults put a good deal of value on words, seeing language development as vitally linked to cognitive development. These adults also see words as critical for social-emotional development. They teach children to use words for problem solving and to express feelings. In a conflict situation, in many programs, you can almost count on some adult saying to the children, "Use your words!" Words are even linked to creativity. For example, when presented with a freshly painted picture, the verbally oriented adult is apt to say, even to the toddler, "Tell me about it."

This approach is very different from expecting the child to learn by being around adults but not being spoken to directly very often. According to Mistry, adults using a nonverbal approach "may model or demonstrate a particular behavior as the child watches...the nonverbal style teaches them to watch and pick up appropriate behavior from their caregivers."[10]

DEFUSING A CROSS-CULTURAL ENCOUNTER

Much of this chapter has focused on comparing what have been called "developmentally appropriate" practices with other practices.[11]

After studying how to work most effectively with young children (all of which is culturally based), we carry a standard. When we meet someone who doesn't fit under that standard, we're disappointed because we expect that person to be like us.[12] For example, when we see how a parent seems to ignore her baby or expect his four year old to behave in an adult environment, that may trigger a reaction. Most of us are conditioned from infancy to think that everyone is like us. Several things can happen when two people with different ideas about the right way to behave meet.

They can both encounter an unpleasant situation or a series of them. Their reaction to the discomfort they feel can be self-protection and withdrawal. This can become a pattern of evasion, which means the two will learn less and less about each other. All this can happen beneath the awareness of either party.

Craig Storti, in *The Art of Crossing Cultures*, suggests a model for changing that pattern. It has to do with first becoming aware of your reaction to behavior that is different from your own. It is important to focus on the feelings as they arise in a cross-cultural encounter and identify them. Reflect on why you are experiencing these feelings because, according to Storti, the mind can't hold two things at once. When you focus on the awareness you dispel the feeling.[13]

Only when the feelings subside can you truly experience what is going on. The more you react, the less you see and hear. Everything is colored by your reactions. Until you quit reacting, you can't truly *experience* something.

This awareness of reactions is not easy. We've been conditioned over a lifetime to have feelings but not to observe them. If you find it hard to develop instant awareness, you can start with retrospective awareness. Look back on the agitated moment and reflect on it. With enough practice, you can eventually bring your awareness process closer to the critical incident that triggered the feelings.

The point is that your first reaction to a certain behavior colors subsequent reactions. The "count-to-ten" approach to anger works in cross-cultural exchanges. Give yourself time; give the other person time. It is often best to stop talking about a disputed issue until everybody has had time to reflect on their initial reactions.

I remember a significant argument regarding whether or not to push children on swings. The staff was divided. The unofficial spokesperson for the hands-off side made the point that children need to learn to swing by themselves. Until they can, she argued, they aren't old enough to use the swings. She was willing to let children lay on their stomachs on the swing and use their feet to move themselves back and forth. Her response triggered a reaction from the other side, which had strong feelings about the proper way to use a swing. "Swings are for sitting!" As the argument escalated, it became obvious that the instant reactions were not helping one side hear the other. Both parties agreed to resume discussion at a future meeting. The cooling-off period helped. The next time the issue was discussed, both sides were able to be more sensitive listeners. If you can step aside from your own reactions, you can begin to understand and respect the behavior of someone who is different from you. You may never come to approve of that behavior; after all, you probably don't approve of everything in your own culture either. But by learning to open yourself up more, you broaden your view and have a better chance of getting along with people different from yourself. Most important, *if you are in a power position, you are less likely to wield your power in ways that inhibit the other person.*

CONCLUSION

Whether adults regard play as valuable and how they plan for and facilitate it may be determined by culture. Disagreements often center around the themes of people versus object orientation, the role of choice, adult involvement in children's play, and emphasis or deemphasis on verbal means of communication.

Adults influence children's learning during play by either valuing it or not, by the environment they choose, by the way they interact in this environment, and by the way they expose children to language. They also influence children by whether or not they present toys, equipment, and materials and by what kind they present.

Some adults think children should be the center of focus in a carefully set up environment. Others think that children should be out of the spotlight and side-line observers in the adult world. Still others think that children's roles should go beyond observation and that they can learn to help and be involved in the adult world.

Some adults think that young children should play only with toys or cast-off household objects (margarine cartons, for example)—things specially designated for them. If children pick up an adult tool, the adult is likely to take it out of their hands, announcing, "That's not a toy!" These adults are likely to childproof the environment, taking the responsibility for keeping children safe.

Other adults let children be part of the adult environment, use adult tools, and learn what is safe and what is not. These adults may or may not provide child toys.

These are very different approaches and present potential conflicts as adults from one orientation collide with those from another.

Naturally, we each think our culture and our values are the right ones. If you're in a position of power with this attitude, it is imperative that you *avoid seeing your job as remediation* when you cross cultures.

Think seriously about what your purpose is in everything you do with young children. Go beyond the cognitive, psychomotor, affective goals you may be used to conceptualizing, and think about what cultural messages you're sending. That's important if you are to become sensitive to cultural differences—tuning in on your own cultural messages.

Ask yourself how you react when a child needs help. Do you take over, or do you facilitate the child's own problem-solving process? Do you respond verbally or nonverbally? How does the manner in which you respond relate to your cultural goals or values?

Be open and humble. No matter how much you know, there's always more to learn.

FOR FURTHER READING

Bergen, Doris, ed., *Play as a Medium for Learning and Development.* Portsmouth, N.H.: Heinemann, 1988. Looks at the benefits of play for children.

Heath, Shirley Brice, *Ways with Words: Language, Life and Work In Communities and Classrooms.* Cambridge: Cambridge University Press, 1983. Fascinating book about language differences and play modes of the groups she studied.

Lubeck, Sally, *The Sandbox Society: Early Education in Black and White America.* Philadelphia: The Falmer Press, 1985. Contrasts African-American and White views of preschool curricula and practices.

Mistry, Jayanthi, "Culture and Learning in Infancy," in Mangione, Peter, ed., *Infant/Toddler Caregiving: A Guide to Culturally Sensitive Care.* Sacramento, Calif.: Far West Laboratory and California Department of Education, 1995. Explains the cultural view that children learn by observing adults, not by playing.

Monighan Nourot, Patricia, Scales, Barbara, Van Horn, Judith and Almy, Milly, *Looking at Children's Play: A Bridge Between Theory and Practice.* New York: Teachers College Press, 1987. Play theory and practice plus more about the benefits.

NOTES

1. Ross, Allen C. (Ehanamani), *Mitakuye Oyasin: We Are All Related.* Denver: Wichoni Waste, 1989, 49–50.

    Dorothy Lee compares cultures that have different concepts of space and time and the implications for emphasizing either activity or silence. She says that Western culture believes "space is empty and to be occupied with matter; time is empty and to be filled with activity. In both primitive and civilized non-Western cultures, on the other hand, free space and time have being and integrity [These cultures have the] conception of nothingness as somethingness....In such societies, children are raised to listen to silence as well as sound. Luther Standing Bear, describing his childhood as an Oglala Dakota in the eighteen-seventies, wrote: 'Children were taught to sit still and enjoy it. They were taught to use their organs of smell, to look when apparently there was nothing to see, and to listen intently when all seemingly was quiet.'...The Wintu Indians have a suffix to refer to alert non-activity, to a silent, non-mobile commitment to awareness....In Japanese traditional culture, free time and space are perceived as the *ma,* the valid interval or meaningful pause." Lee, Dorothy, *Freedom and Culture.* Englewood Cliffs, N.J.: Prentice-Hall, 1959, p. 55.

    According to Thoman and Browder, Chinese Taoist philosophy has a term, "wu wei," which means "nonaction" or "let be." This term implies total passivity, but that's not what it means because the Chinese have no concept of total passivity. Instead they believe that people are always engaged in one of two kinds of activity—going with the flow of the true nature of reality or going against it. Those who look passive are not; they are just refraining from activity that is contrary to nature. Thoman, Evelyn B., and Browder, Sue, *Born Dancing.* New York: Harper and Row, 1987, p. 75.

2. The video "Preschool in Three Cultures" is available from Yale University Press, 92A Yale Station, New Haven, Conn. 06520. Tobin, Joseph J., Wu, David Y. H., and Davidson, Dana H., *Preschool in Three Cultures.* New Haven, Conn.: Yale University Press, 1989.

3. Young, V. H., "Family and Childhood in a Southern Negro Community," *American Anthropologist* 72, 1970, 269–288.

    Young, V. H. "A Black American Socialization Pattern," *American Ethnologist* 1, 1974, 405–413.

4. Mistry, Jayanthi, "Culture and Learning in Infancy: Implications for Caregiving," in *Infant/Toddler Caregiving: A Guide to Culturally Sensitive Care*, Jesus Cortez and Carol Lou Young-Holt, eds. Sacramento: California Department of Education, 1995, p. 21.

5. Hsu, Francis L. K., *Americans and Chinese: Purpose and Fulfillment in Great Civilizations.* Garden City, N.Y.: Natural History Press, 1970, pp. 84–85.

6. Ehling, Marta Borbon, "The Mexican American (El Chicano)," in *Culture and Childrearing*, A. L. Clark, ed. Philadelphia: F. A. Davis, 1981, p. 197.

7. Mistry, "Culture and Learning in Infancy," p. 26.

8. Hall, Edward T., *Beyond Culture.* Garden City, N.Y.: Anchor Press/Doubleday, 1981, pp. 104–116.

9. Heath, S. B., *Ways with Words: Language, Life, and Work in Communities and Classrooms.* Cambridge: Cambridge University Press, 1983.

10. Mistry, "Culture and Learning in Infancy," p. 23.

11. Bredekamp, Sue, ed., *Developmental Appropriate Practice in Early Childhood Programs Serving Children from Birth Through Age 8.* Washington, D.C.: National Association for the Education of Young Children, 1987.

12. According to Storti, "We assume that others are like us for the simple reason that we learned to behave by watching and imitating them. This is the process of conditioning through which we learn how to function in the world: By observing, imitating (for which we are rewarded) and eventually internalizing the behavior of those around us....Thus, while we may not choose to assume that others are like us, while we may even *know* better than to assume that others are like us, and while we may very much wish we could stop expecting everyone to be like us, the force of our conditioning leaves us no alternative." Storti, Craig, *The Art of Crossing Cultures.* Yarmouth, Maine: Intercultural Press, 1990, pp. 49–50.

13. Ibid.

CHAPTER SEVEN

Socialization

We are socialized to look at ourselves, the world, and our role in it, in certain ways. We socialize the children according to the way we were socialized. I was taught that I am an individual. I perceive that I am made to stand on my own two feet—both literally and figuratively. I see myself as separate and different from other people.

As an individual, it's up to me to make a place for myself in this world. I was taught that I was special, and was encouraged to show my "specialness." Likewise, I tried to make each child that I worked with in my early childhood programs feel special.

Now I know that every culture doesn't stress individuality. Some cultures see a strong interconnectedness that regards the individual as unimportant. When I read about "interconnectedness," I still think of individuals as being separate people enmeshed in webs of attachments. But that's not what some people mean. They mean that there's a oneness that isn't made up of separate individuals but of parts of a whole. This view is a very different way to perceive the world and people in general—a view I'm just beginning to understand.[1]

The idea of standing out from the crowd is undesirable for some who see people as part of something bigger. The separateness and flaunting of one's individuality is frowned on by these people. Look at how these themes play out in the following day-care setting:

> You're a caregiver in an infant-toddler center that is part of a larger preschool day-care program. You're the only staff member of your culture, but more than half of the families the program serves are of the same culture as you. One day you find yourself confronting the whole staff at an in-service training on self-esteem when the hired

consultant who is conducting the training uses the phrase "stand out as a unique individual" once too often. Suddenly you find yourself rising out of your seat and speaking passionately to the group. You say, "I'm sick of hearing our children called unique individuals, and I don't think they should stand out!"

The other staff members turn in their seats and stare at you, surprised to hear you express your opinion in this bold manner. You suddenly sit back down and lower your eyes.

The consultant, who is looking at you with all the rest, says quietly, "Go on. Tell us what you mean."

"Well," you start hesitantly, "in my family, we don't keep telling the children that they are special and unique all by themselves. We tell them that they are a member of our family—of our people. Of course they are unique, but their uniqueness makes them fit in—not stand out. They each have something to contribute—not for themselves, but for us all."[2]

"I see you have some strong feelings about this." The consultant leads you on, allowing you to discover where you are going with it.

"I sure do," you find yourself saying. "In this program, we're constantly hammering in the message about it's good to find your identity by standing alone—being an individual. Take all this business about the names in children's clothes and making a big fuss about what belongs to whom. I get sick of that. You're teaching the children the importance of private possessions—ownership. I see sharing as much more important. Otherwise the children grow up to be selfish and too attached to their own things and eventually tend to view them as special and unique just like they are—a further way to make them stand out."

You think you're finished until the consultant shushes a staff member who is about to argue with you, turns to you again, and says, "Anything else on your mind?"

You suddenly realize you're not through as another torrent of words comes pouring out, and you find yourself saying, "I hate the way we're told to praise the children for each little accomplishment. It's like putting a spotlight on them for their individualism. Personally, I detest being in a spotlight."[3] Suddenly you're quiet as you realize how uncomfortable you feel about what's happening right now. You're not only in the spotlight, but you're expressing a personal opinion—just like the unique individuals you've been criticizing. You feel torn apart until you remember that you're not doing it for yourself; you're doing it for all the parents of the children in your center who either don't know about the cultural differences their little ones are experiencing or know about them but haven't felt comfortable questioning the "experts."

"You don't believe in pride?" One staff member overrides the silence the consultant has put on the rest of the group.

Without thinking, you jump back in again. "Sure I believe in pride—but not personal pride. I can't stand to see children go around oozing out the message, 'I'm so great, look at me, pay attention to how wonderful and special I am.'"

"Say more about your ideas about pride," the consultant urges.

"Well, we should help the children feel proud of being a member of the group, praise them when they care about each other. We could do a lot more to get them to help one another than we do. We're all so busy getting them to be unique individuals that they're turning into selfish little brats."

"Why didn't you ever say any of this before?" The director breaks in, again overriding the silence the consultant has imposed on the group so you could get your say in.

"Because one time I did—not here, at another program. I was told that I was wrong. I was told that this is America, and people who live here should think and act like Americans—when in Rome and all that stuff. I was so mad I couldn't even answer. I'm an American. Some people in my family were here a long time ago—even before the English speakers came. Others in my family have come more recently, but most people in America have come from somewhere else anyway. What makes them more American than me?"

Once the flood gates were opened, the water stayed stirred up for quite a while. Eventually, a number of sensitively led discussions brought everyone's feelings and views out into the open. At the staff meetings, a greater number of voices began to express a wider diversity of opinions than had been heard before. As a result, most of the staff gained a larger perspective. The staff continued to work on being more sensitive to cultural and individual differences in the center where this scene occurred. It took a lot of arguments and difficult feelings to get to the place where the staff agreed to disagree. Most finally came to believe that because one person disagrees with another doesn't mean one is right and the other wrong, only that they have different perspectives.

THE SOCIALIZATION PROCESS

The socialization process through which children learn to get along with others starts at birth. Through it, children come to see themselves in relationship to those around them and eventually to the wider society. The goals parents have for the socialization of their children depend on their culture and their value systems (individual, familial, and cultural). The goals a program has may or may not mesh with each parent's goals. This chapter examines where goals, and the values behind them, may clash and what to do about the conflicts that arise.

SAMPLE CONFLICTS

The conflict illustrated by the previous scene deals with the concept of a person as an individual. The white, European-based, Canadian and U.S. cultures look at a child, starting at birth, as a person who must be helped to recognize that he or she is separate and distinct from any other human being. The child is perceived to have an identity, rights, and needs starting at the moment of birth. Because the child is not born with the concept of being a separate individual, one of the goals of the early months is to shatter the newcomer's belief that he or she and the universe are one.

One of the rights of an individual is the right to privacy (also called a need), which is a big issue for members of "individualistic" cultures. Parents go to some trouble to arrange for their privacy. They carry this over to the infant, sending the message that privacy is important. One problem many see with typical child care arrangements in this country is that babies and toddlers lack privacy due to the numbers of children and the need for all to be under close supervision. Provision is sometimes made for nooks and crannies to serve as "hideaways" for children in day care.

There is also some worry about children in child care coming to see themselves as individuals with possessions because what they use at the center belongs to the program, not to individual children.[4]

Not all cultures are "individualistic." In fact, in some, the "self" is not conceived as something apart, separate from others. The smallest unit is the group, of which individuals are a part rather than wholes in themselves.[5] Children in these cultures are taught to see themselves as part of something larger than themselves: their family, their people.

Of course, independence as an individual and the ability to function as a group member are not mutually exclusive; every culture depends on both. But in some cultures, the former has the greater priority, and in other cultures, the latter does.

When these two systems—an individual-oriented system and a group-oriented system—bump up against each other, sparks may fly. One of the most important sentences people who find themselves in an argument over perceptions, beliefs, concepts, or values can learn to use is this one: **"I'm not saying you're wrong; I'm just saying I disagree with you."**

OTHER AREAS OF CONFLICT

Possessions

Just as babies must learn to differentiate themselves from others in cultures that place importance on the individual, toddlers must differentiate between what is theirs and what is not. One of the primary tasks of toddlerhood is learning to think in terms of private property.

Some cultures have a different view of private possessions. Francis Hsu says of the Chinese culture:

> Not only do parents have freedom of action with reference to the children's belongings, but the youngsters can also use the possessions of the parents if they can lay their hands on them. If children damage their parents' possessions they are scolded, not

because they touched things that were not theirs but because they are too young to handle them with proper care.[6]

Some cultures put little emphasis on possession and ownership, indeed, on objects in general. They have other priorities. The lessons they teach about touching or not touching, respecting the property of others, are different from those of parents whose possessions are important to them, are part of their identity. These parents who are not object oriented do not teach pride in ownership or consumerism. Of course, any children who watch television get constant messages about consumerism whether their parents believe in it or not. Here are some sample conflicts between adults that can result from differing attitudes about possessions:

1. Arguments regarding what happens to things that are brought from home. Are they to be distinguished from what belongs to the program? Do they stay in a cubby all day? Do they get used or played with but the owner is in charge? Do they get thrown in with everything else?

2. Issues about respecting the property of others. (For example, one child taking another child's lunch.)

3. Attitudes about lost items. (One adult may be very concerned if clothing, toys, or shoes are missing but another adult may not be as concerned.)

4. Children learning consumerism from other children. (Highlighted when a program has "show and tell," during which time children brag about their possessions.)

5. Issues about taking care of things. (For example, children using puzzle pieces as treasure, putting them in purses, and taking them outside to bury them in the sandbox.)

6. Storing things. An object-oriented person may be more concerned about putting things away with all their parts neatly sorted and stored.

Comparing Children

One aspect of socializing children is to teach them to compare themselves with other children. Perhaps most adults don't teach this lesson outright, but because they constantly do it themselves, they model comparison as a way of looking at people. Very often when two adults are discussing a child and one begins to talk of gross motor milestones achieved, the other asks how old the child was or is. This constant comparison of children to each other or to "the charts" develops a certain mind-set in the children, and they pick up the message that comparison means something is better than something else. They learn early that some parents and early childhood educators think that "faster is better."

Not every culture is so comparison minded. Dorothy Lee talks of several cultures that don't stress achievement or indulge in comparisons:

> Navajo adults and children are valued for their sheer being, just because they *are*. There is no urge toward achievement; no one has to strive for success....The Wintu [native Californians] are people who do not compare individuals with one another, or against a standard....For the Lovedue of South Africa...there was no expectation of achievement to be met. Children grew at their own pace, and were allowed to differ as they pleased; they were not assessed against an average. The freedom to follow one's own bent was not endangered by comparison of one child to another as to attainments, physical size or abilities.[7]

Expression of Feelings

When children are regarded as individuals, they may be encouraged to express their feelings. Good early childhood practice says that adults are to accept all feelings as valid and teach appropriate expression of those feelings to children.

Some practitioners see the importance of a child completely exploring a feeling, such as rage. They allow the child to "work it through," regarding what is happening as a process that should not be interrupted until it is finished. Otherwise the unexpressed feelings may remain unfelt and go underground, popping up again and again as leftovers rather than feelings that are entirely connected to the situation that arises. These early childhood practitioners want to reassure the child that expression of feelings won't result in abandonment.

Other cultures don't have the same view of feelings and their expression. They are more concerned about group harmony than about individual expression of, say, anger or fear.

Jerome Kagan says:

> Americans place greater value on sincerity and personal honesty than on social harmony. But in many cultures—Java, Japan, and China, for example—the importance of maintaining harmonious social relationships, and of adopting a posture of respect for the feelings of elders and of authority, demands that each person not only suppress anger but, in addition, be ready to withhold complete honesty about personal feelings in order to avoid hurting another. This pragmatic view of honesty is regarded as a quality characteristic of the most mature adult and is given not the derogatory labels of insincerity or hypocrisy.[8]

Dorothy Lee says of the Hopi, "It is his duty to be happy, for the sake of the group, and a mind in conflict and full of anxiety brings disruption, ill-being, to the social unit."[9]

Trinh Ngoc Dung says that in Vietnamese families, "Children are taught at an early age to control their emotions."[10]

It sounds as though the mandate is to repress feelings, a situation that is regarded as unhealthy in white, northern European-derived Canadian and U.S. cultures. But there are other views, like that of Francis Hsu, who compares the prominence of emotions in the American way of life...with the tendency of the Chinese to underplay all matters of the heart....Being individual-centered, the American moves toward social and psychological isolation. His happiness tends to be unqualified ecstasy just as his sorrow is likely to mean unbearable misery. A strong emotionality is inevitable since the emotions are concentrated in one individual.

Being more situation-centered, the Chinese is inclined to be socially or psychologically dependent on others, for this situation-centered individual is tied closer to his world and his fellow men. His happiness and his sorrow tend to be mild since they are shared."[11]

DISCIPLINE

The part of the socialization process that receives the most attention is called discipline. Discipline (guidance) is a much talked about subject among parents and early childhood practitioners. There is great potential for conflict when one adult disciplines or "guides" the child of another, as happens in child care. What follows is an example of a major area of disagreement.

Internalized Versus Externalized Controls

Good early childhood practice, much of which is influenced by the value systems of white Canadians and Americans with northern European backgrounds, dictates that any discipline measure has behind it a goal of self-discipline. In other words, the adult starts, sometime in toddlerhood, guiding and controlling behavior using methods that will lead eventually to the child guiding and controlling his or her own behavior. Though the adult starts with externalized controls, the idea is that they will lead to "inner controls," a term often used by early childhood practitioners.

In some cultures, however, externalized controls are not expected to lead to inner controls.[12] Children are always watched—not just by their parents, but by the whole community. A misbehaving child away from home will be guided and directed by whoever is around. The responsibility for child rearing is shared among the group, and everyone becomes a substitute parent when the occasion arises.[13] According to Lonnie R. Snowden,

[T]he Black community invests effective responsibility for control of children's behavior in an extensive network of adults....Because of this extended parenting, children's behavior receives proper monitoring and more immediate sanctions than is the norm in American society. Children may be expected to develop more active exploratory tendencies and assertive styles, since respected external agencies can be counted on to reliably check excess. The school, however, exercises less direct and legitimate control, while expecting a relatively docile, immobile pattern of behavior. The cultural conflict is clearly drawn.[14]

How difficult it is when adults expect children to behave as if the locus of control lies within them. Not many adults expect this of infants or toddlers, but they expect it of preschoolers. If they discipline with the idea of eventual inner controls in mind, the methods they use may be quite different from adults who see the locus of control as something external to the child. Gone is the kind of cultural consistency that empowers the child.

Sandoval and De La Roza describe the way extended family and interdependent network orientation work to provide external controls in the Hispanic community:

> In grocery stores and other public places the mother is not inhibited from shouting directives to the young children to constantly remind them—even when engaged in no mischief—that her inquiring but protective eyes are on them....By loudly verbalizing their directives they also mean to engage others in the social control of their children, seeking a sort of consensus protection. [If I (the mother) were to see other children getting into trouble I would tend to them as if they were my own.][15]

It's not too hard to see what kind of problems might arise for children who are disciplined one way at home and another way in child care. When no one gives children "directives," as in the previous example, do they wonder if no one cares what they do? That would be a strange feeling indeed. If teachers become dedicated to the idea that being fair doesn't mean treating all children the same, they will be able to expand their notions of guidance. Once they know that a child is more used to external control messages, teachers can pay attention to what those messages are and learn to watch closely, use eye contact, and send various signals more like the kind of authority the child is used to.

Cynthia Ballenger, in her article "Because You Like Us: The Language of Control," discusses a contrast between the mainstream North American early childhood educators' ways of managing behavior and Haitian ways. "The North American teachers are concerned with making a connection with the individual child, with articulating his or her feelings and problems." North Americans use consequences as an explanation of why not to do something. Nothing is good or bad in itself, but behavior has consequences. The child must learn about each situation. Consequences are the issue, not shared morals and values.

Instead of referring to feelings or consequences, Haitian teachers "emphasize the group in their control talk, articulating the values and responsibilities of group membership." They don't differentiate specific behaviors, but lump everything into "bad behavior." Haitian adults are clear about good and bad, and so are their children. The children know why they need to be good: so they don't bring shame on their families. It's a system of shared values. The lessons are taught in a question-and-answer format. "Do your parents let you kick?" The children understand their role and repeat the expected answers. The sequence often ends with a statement like, "When an adult talks to you, you're supposed to listen so you will become a good person. The adults here like you, they want you to become good children."

Ballenger uses the example of herself helping children cross a parking lot to show "Haitian control talk."

CINDY: "Did I tell you to go?"

CHILDREN: "No."

CINDY: "Can you cross this parking lot by yourselves?"

CHILDREN: "No."

CINDY: "That's right. There are cars here. They're dangerous. I don't want you to go alone. Why do I want you to wait for me?

CLAUDETTE: "Because you like us."

Even though Ballenger was using the cultural style familiar to the children, she expected a response about consequences. Instead, she got an answer more like Haitian ways. Ballenger says that, in the Haitian way, a reprimand defines and strengthens relationships.

This statement really hit home with me. I learned long ago in my early childhood training not to scold or reprimand children in any way. I approach disciplinary matters in a positive way. I avoid words like good and bad. I never use love as a reason for doing something. I can get through a whole day in preschool without ever saying "No." I'm not criticizing myself, I'm proud of my skills. However, I admit that my approach may be misinterpreted by children who are used to a more stringent, controlling, and therefore, to them, a more loving approach.[16]

Physical Punishment

Another difference in discipline approaches may be the use of physical punishment rather than explaining, showing disapproval, redirecting, using time out, and a host of other techniques all of which avoid physical punishment. Ugly conflicts can arise over this issue, especially when some adults believe firmly in nonviolence and others believe in the benefits of a good spanking and have never experienced any other way of handling children's behavior.

If, however, you work in an early childhood program of any sort, no matter what your culture, you don't have the choice to use physical punishment because the law forbids it. Further, you're bound by law to report suspected physical abuse (physical punishment that leaves marks on the child). Be sure parents know this from the start so they won't feel betrayed if you have to report suspected abuse.[17] In cases where parents disagree with approaches that avoid physical punishment, it's important to start a dialogue. Be respectful of their differing beliefs, but clear about the law.

Conflicts are bound to arise when children get together. How you handle them reflects your values (which relate to your culture). Here's the typical white, European-American, early childhood practitioner's view: although a reasonable number of conflicts between toddlers provides valuable learning experiences, it's worthwhile to prevent excessive conflicts. Conflict prevention comes through careful arrangement of the environment so one child is less likely to encroach upon another. Plenty of toys and things to do help prevent fights.

When children do get into a conflict, tussling or struggling with each other, the adult comes immediately to the scene to prevent anyone from getting hurt. He or she either settles the problem or gets down on the children's level and talks them through it so they can settle it themselves. Keeping one child from hurting another, even slightly, is an important value for the typical white, European-American, early childhood practitioner.

That value is not universal. As a Japanese teacher says, "As the year progresses we put fewer and fewer toys out during free-play time to give children additional opportunities to learn to share and to deal with the conflicts which arise." Then the teacher stays back and lets the children work out the problem. In fact, one child who continually provoked fights and hurt children was considered to "serve the function of giving other children a chance to experience a range of emotions and to rehearse a variety of strategies both for resolving their own disagreements as well as for mediating conflicts among others."[18]

This approach in the Japanese program provided quite a contrast to Chinese ideas about discipline:

> According to Chinese theories of child development, children are not born knowing how to behave correctly and they are unlikely to come to know correct behavior through unsupervised play with peers or through a process of self-discovery and self-actualization...teachers bear the responsibility of teaching students self-restraint and correct behavior.[19]

POWER AND AUTHORITY

Carol Phillips advises that when you're working across cultures, it is important to know how parents want their children to relate to authority figures.[20]

How the authority figures themselves behave is also an issue that can be of importance. When authority figures—teachers or caregivers in a program—behave differently from the way children are used to, those children can experience cultural dissonance. Janice Hale-Benson says, "Black mothers tend to be more firm and physical in their discipline than white mothers, consequently, when the child encounters a white teacher in school practicing all the techniques she learned in college, the children 'run all over her' and are labeled discipline problems."[21]

Related to authority is power. A word heard more and more in early childhood programs these days is "empowerment." Early childhood practitioners are busy trying to empower children, parents, and each other as they work day to day in centers and family day-care homes across the nation. What does this word mean, and what is the potential for cultural conflicts?

To empower means to bring out the power of the individual or group. Empowerment is based on the idea that power, like love, comes from within and exists in unlimited supply. In fact, the more you empower others, the more you can experience your own personal power. It's not like commodities—when you give away what you have, the other person has not only what he had before but yours besides, and you have nothing. Empowering does not mean giving power up, but rather bringing power out. Empowering has to do with personal power, not with overpowering or controlling others.

Everyone doesn't see power in this way. Imagine the conflicts that can arise when adults have differing views of power and its uses. What does that mean in terms of interacting with the children? Will one adult understand when another is using her own power either *with* the child or *for* the child rather than *over* the child?

Here is an example of two different ways adults might react to a child when they have differing views of power and the adult role in relationship to power.

> Picture a two year old girl trying to solve a problem; she's working to get a toy on a shelf just out of her reach. The adult sitting on the floor nearby is trying to empower her by supporting her in solving this problem without handing her a solution. She waits to see what the child will do. The child continues straining and reaching until she gives up, angry and discouraged. As she moves away from the shelf, she passes by the seated adult, who pushes a large plastic block toward her. Seeing the block was all she needed. Immediately, the child starts shoving it over to the shelf and is about to climb up on it to reach the toy when another caregiver comes over, takes the block away, says, "No, don't climb on that," and walks over to put the block back where it belongs.

You can see the potential for conflict here as one adult defeats the other's purpose and relates to the child in an entirely different way.

When two people or two groups have opposing ways of doing things, one way is not necessarily right and the other way necessarily wrong. The two ways are different, and differences should be respected. One way, especially if it is your own, may feel a lot righter to you. Can you suspend judgment, shift reference frames, and accept that there's another way?

Just because you know something about a person's culture doesn't mean you can predict that person's behavior. Individuals are guided by their individual values, inclinations, behavior styles, and cultural background. Knowing a person's culture tells you something about the probability that he or she will behave in a certain way; it doesn't tell you that he or she *will* behave in that way.

LEARNING TO "READ" INDIRECT COMMUNICATION

This chapter started with a scene of a teacher expressing herself directly from the heart about her disagreements with socialization practices that were in conflict with her values. Was there a slightly fictional tone to that scene? If you felt the tone, it was because it's very unlikely that people from a culture that has that particular set of values would stand up to a crowd and express themselves in that manner.

In order to get feedback from someone who doesn't believe in the "spotlight," who avoids direct confrontation, who feels it's rude to argue, you have to learn to read subtle messages. If you ask directly, you're more likely to find the person telling you what you want to hear than criticizing you or the situation. The primary issue is not honesty but manners and harmony. You may feel irritated that you seem to be expected to read minds. But if you educate yourself a bit, you'll find others who are accustomed to this kind of communication are able to pick up on the subtle verbal and nonverbal messages. It isn't really a matter of reading minds; it's a matter of picking up clues.

Let's go back to the teacher at the beginning of this chapter and look at all the clues she sent out before she reached the point of direct verbal communication. It's important to realize that she acted out of character by directly confronting the entire staff. She reached that point only because she was seeing a European-American therapist who taught her this type of personal expression. Even though she learned to do it, she felt very uncomfortable because such bold criticism went against everything she believed in. (It's more realistic to assume she never would have spoken out so directly, no matter how unhappy or uncomfortable she felt.) But this teacher gave clues to the director long before the staff meeting brought everything to a head.

The first clue came when the teacher complained to a third party about the program, expecting her to deliver the message to the director. She was unhappy about what she considered the cultural inappropriateness of the program's approach to socialization. But the message delivered to the director wasn't stated in those terms. What the third party reported was the teacher's discomfort with a particular incident. This incident wasn't very important in the mind of the director. And the director's reaction to getting the message secondhand was anger. She discounted the whole situation because the teacher hadn't approached her directly. She decided it wasn't worth putting any energy into what she termed "hearsay" and "gossip."

If the director had been more culturally sensitive, she might have seen that third-party communication was a means of avoiding direct confrontation that is perfectly acceptable and even expected by many people.

Another series of clues came when every once in a while the teacher criticized the director's culture in general, but then always exempted anyone of that culture within hearing distance. "But you aren't like that..." she had said more than once to the director. What the director didn't know was that on each of these occasions, the teacher had given her a bit of personal feedback about her own behavior. It was roundabout, but that's the accepted way of the teacher's culture.

The director decided to educate herself, so she asked the teacher to teach her about her culture. Although the director's attitude brought the two closer, unfortunately, it was too big a request. It was hard for the teacher to go beyond the outward, easily recognized elements of her culture. She began educating the director about its art, music, and food. She avoided any direct reference to the nitty-gritty of what was bothering her.

While they were establishing their relationship around manifestations of culture, avoiding important cultural conflicts, the teacher continued giving out subtle messages. The director missed every one of them. During one staff meeting, for example, when they were talking about labeling the children's belongings, the teacher brought up a very feeble objection. No one even understood what she was saying; and when the conversation wandered to another subject, she remained silent. The director went back to pick up on her objection, but by then, the teacher just went along with the majority. The director decided that she had changed her mind. What the director didn't realize was that even just voicing a mild opinion was hard for the teacher. The fact that she spoke up at all indicated she had very strong feelings. But the director, because of her own background, where speaking your mind was the ordinary approach, didn't regard the teacher's mild objection as very important.

Many people, when placed in the director's position, feel frustrated at the least and perhaps quite angry and even lied to when told that messages have been sent but have not been picked up. The indirect means of communication so common among some people are very upsetting to someone of a culture that values straightforwardness and honesty.

It's important if you're in the director's position to try to look at indirect communication not as wrong, bad, or dysfunctional, but as simply *another way* of communicating. You can try to teach your way, but realize that it will be no easier for the other person to change than it is for you to change. Perhaps the most you can hope for is mutual respect and understanding.

To socialize children across cultures, you need to open up communication and get all adults involved to observe what's going on and try to understand how the others feel about it. Maybe you can get things out in the open; but even if you do, it's important to realize that, though you can talk about goals and values, it's how you treat the children, how they react to you, and how you respond back that makes the difference. Only through actions and interactions will differences in goals and values have meaning—otherwise it all remains in the realm of theory.

FOR FURTHER READING

Ballenger, Cynthia, "Because You Like Us: The Language of Control," *Harvard Educational Review* 62(2), Summer 1992, 199–208. Thought-provoking article that contrasts Haitian and North American early childhood professional discipline approaches.

Lee, Fong Yun, "Asian Parents as Partners," *Young Children*, March 1995, 4–8. Discusses the perspective and core values of five Asian cultures.

Little Soldier, Lee, "Working with Native American Children," *Young Children*, September 1992. Information about Native American socialization and how to relate to Native American children in culturally sensitive ways.

Medicine, Beatrice, "Child Socialization Among Native Americans: The Lakota (Sioux) in Cultural Context," *Wicazo Sa Review* 1(2), Fall 1985, 23–28. Helps the reader understand Native American perspectives on socialization.

Ramirez, M., and Castenada, A., *Cultural Democracy, Bicognitive Development and Education*. New York: Academic Press, 1974. A classic book that brought to attention the idea of field-independent and field-sensitive learners.

Rodriguez, R., *The Hunger of Memory: The Education of Richard Rodriguez*. New York: Bantam Books, 1983. A firsthand account of one child's socialization.

Tobin, Joseph J., Wu, David Y. H., and Davidson, Dana H., *Preschool in Three Cultures*, New Haven, CT: Yale University Press, 1989. A thought-provoking look at differences in preschool practices and the values behind them. The study included North American, Chinese, and Japanese preschools and day care.

Wong-Fillmore, Lilly, "When Learning a Second Language Means Losing the First," *Early Childhood Research Quarterly* 6, 1991, 223–229. Explains the serious problems with cultural identification and family relationships that occur when children lose their home language.

NOTES

1. Leslie Willams writes about the Native American perspective that the group is central and says, "The development of the individual is not seen to be as worthy of attention as is the relationship of that individual to the group. The growth of any one person is seen as integrally tied with the health and integrity of the group as a whole. Thus, the focus is not so much on the internal dynamic as on relationship of the self to others—and others can include human beings, other beings (including spiritual entities), and the external, material world. The highlighting of relationship may sometimes mean the subsuming of self for the good and enhancement of others." Williams, Leslie R., "Developmentally Appropriate Practice and Cultural Values: A Case in Point," in Mallory, Bruce L., and New, Rebecca S., eds., *Diversity and Developmentally Appropriate Practices: Challenges for Early Childhood Education*. New York: Teachers College Press, 1994, 160.

Elleni Tedla writes of the notion of interconnection among African people: "The bondedness of everyone in creation is recognized. This awareness of the interconnectedness of fittouran (people) is well expressed in the concepts of diginnet (kindness, generosity, caring). Tedla, Elleni, *Sankofa: African Thought and Education.* New York: Peter Lang, 1995.

The title of A. C. Ross's book, *Mitakuye Oyasin (We Are All Related),* shows his emphasis on the subject in the Lakota tradition. Ross, Allen C. (Ehanamani), *Mitakuye Oyasin: We Are All Related.* Denver: Wichoni Waste, 1989.

2. Many writers and researchers discuss the contrasting concepts of a person as an individual versus a person as a part of a group. Hall speaks of those Americans who, like himself, regard the individual as a meaningful concept: "We draw a line around the individual and say this is our basic entity—the building block of all social relations and institutions....None of this can be applied to the Pueblo Indian for something akin to lineages in the Pueblo are the viable unit. No human being outside of these groups has significance independent and distinct from the group. The Pueblo view of the group as the basic unit is difficult if not impossible for the average European to comprehend, because he lacks the experience of having grown up in such a group." Hall, Edward T., *Beyond Culture.* Garden City, N.Y.: Anchor Press/Doubleday, 1981, p. 231.

Tobin et al., in discussing the research done through comparing videotapes of early childhood programs in three countries, say, "Virtually all the Japanese preschool teachers who viewed our tape of an American preschool contrasted the individualism they perceive as characterizing preschool in America with the groupism they believe characterizes their own society and schools." But according to the teachers who commented on the tapes, the goal wasn't to get everybody doing the same thing at the same time. "That isn't the same as real group life....We just try to show them, to teach them the fun and sense of belonging one can get only by being part of a group." No longer are duty and sacrifice foremost values. The teachers' stated goals involved achieving a balance between individualism and groupism: "integrate the individual and group dimensions of self." Tobin, Joseph J., Wu, David Y. H., and Davidson, Dana H., *Preschool in Three Cultures.* New Haven, Conn: Yale University Press, 1989, pp. 71, 38–40.

Hsu says, "In the American way of life the emphasis is placed upon the predilections of the individual, a characteristic we shall call *individual-centered.* This is in contrast to the emphasis the Chinese put upon an individual's appropriate place and behavior among his fellowmen, a characteristic we shall term *situation centered.*" Hsu, Francis L. K., *Americans and Chinese: Purpose and Fulfillment in Great Civilizations.* Garden City, N.Y.: Natural History Press, 1970, p. 10.

Lubeck discusses two distinct cultural patterns: "A collective orientation is apparent when enculturation occurs in a shared function environment where the focus is on social relations, stressing 'kinship,' interdependency, and cooperation, a holistic world view, relational thinking, and the importance of non-verbal communication. An individualistic orientation predominates when enculturation occurs in a nucleated family structure, focusing on manipulatory experience and stressing self-achievement, competition, the ability to abstract parts from wholes, abstract thinking and the importance of verbal communication." Lubeck, Sally, *Sandbox Society: Early Education in Black and White America.* Philadelphia: Falmer Press, 1985, p. 110.

Holtzman says, "Mexicans tend to be more family-centered, while Americans are more individual-centered." Holtzman, Wayne H., Diaz-Guerrero, Rogelio, and Swartz, Jon D., *Personality Development in Two Cultures: A Cross-Cultural Longitudinal Study of School Children in Mexico and the United States.* Austin: University of Texas Press, 1975, p. 359.

Suzuki laments the deculturalization of Asian-American life. He argues that the institutions of education and mental health have mistakenly failed to realize the successes of Asian-American child-rearing in inculcating family values that may run counter to the accepted norm in terms of individualism and aggressiveness. Suzuki, Bob H., The Asian-American Family," in *Parenting in a Multicultural Society*, Mario D. Fantini and René Cardenas, eds. New York: Longman, 1980, pp. 97–98.

3.   A number of cultures shy away from spotlighting children for their individual accomplishments. Dorothy Lee has this to say about the Hopis on this subject: "The Hopis have a reluctance to stand out, to be singled out from the group. Teachers in Hopi schools have reported discomfort and even tears as a reaction to praise in public. It appears that what is in fact disturbing is the comparative evaluation that results in singling out and praising. Hopi do not compare their achievement, nor the importance of their work." Lee, Dorothy, *Freedom and Culture.* Englewood Cliffs, N.J.: Prentice-Hall, 1959, p. 20.

"Southeast Asian cultural attitudes toward 'singling out' any individual in their society as being 'different' in any way…are literally worlds apart from expectations prevalent in the United States." Morrow, Robert D., "Cultural Differences—Be Aware!" *Academic Therapy* 23(2), November 1987, p. 143.

"Modesty and humility for Vietnamese are important social graces, and deeply ingrained into their identity." Duong Thanh Binh, *A Handbook for Teachers of Vietnamese Students: Hints for Dealing with Cultural Differences in Schools.* Arlington, Vir.: Center for Applied Linguistics, 1975, p. 16.

Amy Tan points out that an issue in Chinese character development is "how to know your own worth and polish it, never flashing it around like a cheap ring." Tan, Amy, *The Joy Luck Club.* New York: Putnam's, 1989, p. 254.

4.   Dorothy Lee discusses the relationship of freedom, possessions, and privacy in "individualistic" cultures. "The child grows up needing time to himself, a room of his own, freedom of choice, freedom to plan his own time and his own life. He will brook no interference and no encroachment. He will spend his wealth installing private bathrooms in his house, buying a private car, a private yacht, private woods, and a private beach, which he will then people with his privately chosen society. The need for privacy is an imperative one in our society, recognized by official bodies of our government. And it is part of a system which stems from and expresses our basic value." Lee, *Freedoom and Culture*, p. 74.

5.   "Traditional Asian American-Pacific American culture differs from western cultures in that Asians tend to place great emphasis on the family as the central unit rather than the individual." Root, Maria, Ho, Christine, and Sue, Stanley, "Issues in the Training of Counselors for Asian Americans," in *Cross-Cultural Training for Mental Health Professionals*, H. Lefley and P. Pedersen, eds. Springfield, Ill.: Charles C. Thomas, 1986, p. 202.

According to Caudill and his associates, his research showed that the Caucasian-American mother was more "individual oriented and independent….She saw her infant from birth as a separate and autonomous individual with his own needs and desires....In contrast the motherland Japanese mother was observed to be more group oriented and interdependent in her relations....The Japanese-American mothers...appeared to be somewhere in between." Sodetani-Shibata, Aimee Emiko, "The Japanese American," in *Culture and Childrearing*, A. L. Clark, ed. Philadelphia: F. A. Davis, 1981, p. 121.

Hmong society is extremely group oriented, with the family being the most important social unit. Matthiessen, Neba, *The Hmong: A Multicultural Study*. Fairfield, Calif.: Fairfield-Suisun Unified School District, 1987.

Children "are taught to be loyal first to their family, to consider the wishes of the family over their own." Trinh Ngoc Dung, "Understanding Asian Families: A Vietnamese Perspective," *Children Today*, March–April 1984, p. 12.

"In the U.S. we begin early to groom our children to become independent. We stress early weaning, dressing and feeding oneself at the preschool level, thinking for yourself, being your 'own person,' and becoming self-sufficient children and adults. Almost as soon as an American child is born, he sleeps by himself, often in his own bedroom. Toys and other possessions are identified as 'mine' or 'yours.' American parents foster self-reliance, assertiveness, speaking one's mind, and looking out for 'number one.'

"With Southeast Asians, the opposite is true...in contrast to the American emphasis on egocentric, independent behavior, the Southeast Asian child is trained to think of the family first and must learn to subjugate his own personal desires and concerns." Morrow, "Cultural Differences," p. 144.

6. Hsu, *Americans and Chinese*, pp. 75, 84–85.

7. Lee, *Freedom and Culture*, pp. 10, 51.

8. Kagan, Jerome, *The Nature of the Child*. New York: Basic Books, 1984, pp. 244–245.

9. Lee, *Freedom and Culture*, p. 21.

10. Trinh, "Understanding Asian Families," p. 12.

11. Hsu, *Americans and Chinese*, p. 10.

12. External controls aren't just a way to guide behavior in childhood. Even in adulthood, for some cultures, the expectation is that external controls are still needed. Hall gives us an example: "in the northern European tradition until very recently, sexual controls were vested in the woman for the most part; i.e., internalized. In southern Europe this was not so. The controls were in the situation (people) and in physical structures (doors and locks). For years, people in middle- and upper-class Latin America believed that the sexual drive was so strong in men and the capacity of women to resist was so weak, that if a man and a woman were alone together behind closed doors neither could be expected to be able to resist the overwhelming power of the man's drive. Walls, doors, and locks were a physical extension of morality— externalizations of process handled internally by middle-class North Americans." Hall, *Beyond Culture*, p. 27.

13. Janice Hale-Benson reports: "adults in the Black community play substantially different roles as social control agents than do adults in the school...a network of significant adults firmly corrects undesirable behavior whenever it occurs and report such behavior to the parent. Therefore, parents are at the center of this social control network. For the child, this means that he is always under the surveillance of adults.

The significant feature of the control system is that it seems to operate external to the child. Therefore, the child seems to develop external locus of control.

"In the school situation, adults seem to behave as if locus of social control exists within the child. They do not function in ways that are consistent with the child's expectations of how adults should behave toward them in situations that require the enforcement of social controls." Hale-Benson, Janice E., *Black Children: Their Roots, Culture, and Learning Styles*. Baltimore: Johns Hopkins University Press, 1986, p. 85.

14. Snowden, Lonnie R., "Toward Evaluation of Black Psycho-Social Competence," in *The Pluralistic Society*, Stanley Sue and Thom Moore, eds. New York: Human Sciences Press, 1984, p. 188.

15. Sandoval, M., and De La Roza, M. "A Cultural Perspective for Serving the Hispanic Client," in *Cross-Cultural Training for Mental Health Professionals*, Harriet Lefley and Paul Pedersen, eds. Springfield, Ill.: Charles C. Thomas, 1986, p. 167.

16. Ballenger, Cynthia, "Because You Like Us: The Language of Control," *Harvard Educational Review* 62(2), Summer 1992, 199–208.

17. You may run into some real cultural conflicts over the definitions of child abuse. According to Shwartz, "In the Chinese culture to not physically discipline one's children, using what may be fairly severe means and methods, is seen within the cultural context as deviant....Black and Hispanic parents and professionals like-wise site [sic] the use of spanking and other forms of physical discipline as being part of their child-rearing practices for generations...many lower class white families share similar values around authority and discipline. Hispanic families, especially recent immigrants, are truly shocked at the idea of an agency or the state intervening in their private family life and telling them anything about how they discipline their children. Jorge Santiz, a consultant formerly with the San Francisco Child Abuse council, says, 'Child abuse doesn't exist as a legal concept in most Latin countries.' That a child has legal rights separate from the family that are protected by law is a particularly Western notion, rooted in individualism. In many Asian, Latin, and non-western cultures, filial piety is of much more fundamental value than individualism. The individual is expected to comply with familial authority, to the point of sacrificing one's desires. The already gray area between where a parent's rights end and a child's begins is made all the more murky when value systems as different as these are operating." Shwartz, Deborah, *The Children's Advocate*, January–February 1983, p. 6.

18. Tobin, Wu, and Davidson, *Preschool in Three Cultures*, p. 33.

19. Ibid., p. 96.

20. Phillips, Carol Brunson, "Culture: A Process That Empowers," in *Infant/Toddler Caregiving: A Guide to Culturally Sensitive Care*, Jesus Cortez and Carol Lou Young-Holt, eds. Sacramento: California Department of Education, 1995, p. 7.

21. Hale-Benson, *Black Children*, p. 68.

CHAPTER EIGHT

Conclusion

This book is about adults working with children across cultures. It is also about adults relating across cultures to other adults about the children they work with. It is about resolving differences, living with them, gaining from them, and celebrating them. It is about avoiding a deficit model that says when child-rearing practices deviate from what is considered the norm, they are inadequate rather than reflecting competent or adaptive responses. It is about looking at how values influence child-rearing practices. It is about defining the strengths of diverse practices and looking at how they contribute to the survival and enhancement of the group as well as promoting the mental health of the individuals and families. This book is about regarding differences with mutual respect as well as looking at them as sources of strength.

This book is also about resolving conflicts though mutual negotiation and problem solving, through caregiver and parent education. It is about managing or coping with conflicts that can't be resolved through mutual respect and continued communication.

What has not yet been clarified is with which person you will be doing this talking and conflict management. If you view the nuclear family as the primary family model, you probably regard the mother as the person in charge of the children. You may be surprised when working with families who have different family structures. In some families, the mother does not make the decisions regarding the children. It may be the father, the grandmother, or perhaps someone else who is recognized as the "head of the family." Do not assume automatically that the person who brings the child to the program is the one to talk to. Instead, determine who is the decision maker in the family. If a parent cannot make an independent decision, don't expect him or her to discuss or negotiate any procedure concerning the child with you. In some extended families, the older members make all family-related decisions. As a result, be sure to invite more than just the parents to discussions, conferences, meetings, and social gatherings.

None of this is easy. Relating across cultures causes no end of difficulty. Here's an example: Imagine yourself walking into a center and finding the adults scattered around the room, down on the floor with the children. The adults rarely talk to one another or make eye contact. Instead, they are fully focused on the children, talking to them, responding to them, and now and then initiating something like bringing out a new toy or giving a bottle or a diaper change. These adults are consciously doing what the literature tells them is good child development practice. They are also unconsciously reproducing the role of old-fashioned, mainstream, nuclear family housewife—the one who was there for her children, raising them in an isolated fashion.[1] These caregivers carry out the mainstream goal: to focus on one's children, even sacrifice for them, but expect them to become their own person and move away. They are supposed to become independent of their caregivers. That's exactly what will happen to these children—they'll move from the infant-toddler program on into the preschool program, and the ties with caregivers will be severed in most cases, the attachment gone when they "move on." And the caregivers expect this to happen. They may feel sad, but they want the children to move on to the next level, independent of them.

Now imagine yourself walking into a different center. Here the adults are sitting on adult furniture, up from the floor. They are gathered into one area of the room talking to each other. Several hold babies on their laps, but they don't talk directly to them. Their focus is on adults, yet they manage subtly to incorporate the children into their adult world without shifting their focus dramatically every time they do. They seem to know what's going on in the room at every minute though they aren't obviously supervising. They are not doing what is instantly recognized as "good child development practice" (and they may feel guilty about that fact). They are, however, reflecting an upbringing in an extended family with a lot of adults around. They too know that these children will move up to the "preschool room," leaving their caregivers behind. They may not be as reconciled to the severing of the ties as the adults in the first program, who accept the goal of separation as a valid one. They may not be so happy to think of the children becoming independent of them.

If you are the supervisor of both of these programs, how will you feel about the one that doesn't match your own style, your own set of goals, your own beliefs about what's good for babies? Difficulties arise across cultures not only because of differing values, ways of doing things, and beliefs about how things ought to be, but also because people are governed by systems they are unaware of. They are also unable to dissociate themselves from others. Hall, looking at his own problem with dissociation with a particular person that bothered him a lot, says, "I failed to draw a line separating me from him and was treating him as a recalcitrant, somewhat obnoxious, bumbling part of myself that wouldn't behave."[2] Hall also says:

> Theoretically there should be no problem when people of different cultures meet. Things begin, most frequently, not only with friendship and goodwill on both sides, but there is an intellectual understanding that each party has a different set of beliefs, customs, mores, values or what-have-you. The trouble begins when people have to start working together, even on a superficial basis. Frequently, even after years of close association, neither can make the other's system work! People are in and remain in the grip of the cultural type of identification. Without knowing it, they experience the other person as an uncontrollable and unpredictable part of themselves.[3]

To make things work, according to Hall, "two things must be known: first, that there is a system: and second, the nature of that system."[4] The way you find out about your own system is by contrasting it to other systems. You can find these contrasts when some real-life situation triggers a reaction in you. Tune in on your feelings. Become aware of the whole situation. Only then will you begin to understand differences in behavior from one system to the other. We find out the nature of systems in context—in real-life situations.

In child care, we have numerous real-life situations. We are in the position of discovering an enormous amount of information about ourselves and how our systems work. We can begin to see our own system working as other people don't follow the hidden program we regard as sane and normal. That's the wonderful thing about working with people who are different from us—not having unusual or exotic experiences, but gaining the chance to learn about our own systems. We can achieve that awareness only by interacting with others who do not share our systems (that is, members of the opposite sex, different age groups, different ethnic groups, and different cultures). This book focuses on culture, but we all also come in contact with other systems, systems that can teach us about our own once we tune into the differences. When you can see your own system working, you can make better decisions about how to live your life. You can change it to make it work for you.

As a white Anglo-American who, because of living in the United States today, automatically has privilege and power (unearned, I might add), I am far less aware of systems other than my own than people who are on the lower end of the power differential.[5] This is a fact I am just coming to realize, though when I think about what I know as a woman, I can begin to understand it. Just as I know a lot more about male systems than they know about female systems, so do, for example, African-Americans know more about my system than I know about theirs. The less powerful learn about the more powerful as a survival mechanism.[6]

My point here is that some of us have a lot more to learn than others! And while you (and I) are learning about others' systems, let's be careful to understand that people's behavior cannot be predicted by knowing what culture they belong to. People have individual values, personal inclinations, and behavior styles that determine how they will act. Any statement about culture is a generalization and doesn't tell you how an individual in that culture will act. You can see trends, themes, and probabilities by understanding something about a particular culture, but be careful about generalizing that information to individuals.

I believe in the cultures mingling and mixing. Even though I provided examples of the difficulties, have expressed worries about children not becoming part of their own culture by being exposed to a multicultural setting, and have considered the problems of cultural crossing when one cultural group has more power than the other, I still see cultural mix as a potentially positive experience.

When things work well, children in a bicultural or multicultural program grow up to be highly competent people—able to move freely and comfortably with or away from their own people. They feel good about themselves. They fit, and when they find themselves in a situation where they don't fit, they have a better chance of adapting without giving up anything of themselves or their cultures.

My husband is such a bicultural person. He grew up in a bilingual-bicultural setting in Mexico. His family was part of a German community, though he is only one-quarter German. He spoke both German and Spanish from the beginning and has friends and relatives who are monocultural-monolingual Mexican, monocultural-monolingual German, and bicultural, like himself. He was educated in bilingual schools to such an extent that he could as easily have gone to college in Mexico as in Germany (something rarely true of graduates of bilingual education programs in the U.S., unfortunately).

But instead of going to college in either of those countries, he moved to the United States, where he concentrated on acquiring a third culture and language. Because of his early upbringing (I'm convinced), he learned to fit fairly quickly and easily into middle-class Anglo America without giving up too much of himself. Today he moves with equal ease into a group of Germans, Mexicans, Chicanos, Mexican-Americans, or Anglos, speaking their language and using their gestures, facial expressions, body postures, and all other behaviors that convey cultural consistency. Some of this he is aware of; other aspects must be unconscious. Even his name reflects his chameleon like quality; he is called Frank, Fanko, and Pancho by people who know him in various contexts.

As a monocultural person, I look with envy on those whose abilities are so much broader and more developed than my own. But I have my own background advantages. Having been raised in a single-parent, low-income, extended family that struggled to keep a middle-class status, I have a broader view of class differences than some people. But that subject opens enormous doors that are beyond the scope of this book.

So as I end this book, I try to imagine a world in which people of one culture respect those of another culture, different though it may be, a world in which power differential is a thing of the past, where people know and use their personal power for their own good and that of society, a world that is unified, not in bland sameness, but in rich diversity. I think we can begin to reach such a world through the way we care for children—both at home and in child care. My goal in writing this book is to move one small step toward that world.

FOR FURTHER READING

Hall, Edward T., *Beyond Culture*. Garden City, N.Y.: Anchor Books, 1977. All of Hall 's books explain culture and cultural encounters in helpful ways.

McIntosh, Peggy, *White Privilege and Male Privilege: A Personal Account of Coming to See Correspondences Through Work in Women's Studies*. Working Paper No. 189. Wellesley, Mass.: Wellesley College Center for Research on Women, 1988. Looks at the other side of bias—privilege. An eye-opening article for white people.

Phillips, Carol Brunson, "Culture: A Process that Empowers," in Mangione, Peter, ed., *Infant/Toddler Caregiving: A Guide to Culturally Sensitive Care*, Sacramento, Calif.: Far West Laboratory and California Department of Education, 1995. Argues that empowering children is a major reason to deal with cultural issues in early childhood education.

Young, V. H. "A black American socialization patterning." *American Ethnologist* 1, 1974, 405–413. Discusses some real differences in how adults socialize children.

NOTES

1. Lubeck, Sally, *Sandbox Society: Early Education in Black and White America*. Philadelphia: Falmer Press, 1985, p. 40.

2. Hall, Edward T., *Beyond Culture*. Garden City, N.Y.: Anchor Press/Doubleday, 1981, p. 238.

3. Ibid., p. 239.

4. Ibid., p. 51. Hall also says, "What is more, the only way to master either is to seek out systems that are different from one's own and, using oneself as a sensitive recording device, make note of every reaction or tendency to escalate. Ask yourself questions that will help define the state you were in as well as the one you are escalating to. It is impossible to do this in the abstract, because there are too many possibilities; behavior systems are too complex. The rules governing behavior and structure of one's own cultural system can be discovered only in a specific context or real-life situation." Ibid., p. 91.

5. McIntosh, Peggy, "White Privilege and Male Privilege: A Personal Account of Coming to See Correspondences Through Work in Women's Studies," Working Paper No. 189. Wellesley, Mass: Wellesley College Center for Research on Women, 1988.

6. A student of mine once told me about an assignment another teacher had given his class. The students were to write an essay. The men's assignment was to write about what it would be like to be a woman. The women's assignment was to write about what it would be like to be a man. The contrast was startling to everyone. The women wrote reams; the men either failed to turn in the assignment or wrote less than a page. Women know more about men, in general, than the reverse.

Bibliography

Anderson, P., "Explaining Intercultural Differences in Nonverbal Communication," in Samovar, L., and Porter, R., eds., *Intercultural Communication: A Reader.* Belmont, Calif.: Wadsworth, 1994.

Anderson P., and Fenichel, E. S., *Serving Culturally Diverse Families of Infants and Toddlers with Disabilities.* Washington, D.C.: National Center for Clinical Infant Programs, 1989 ED 318174.

Ballenger, Cynthia, "Because You Like Us: The Language of Control." *Harvard Educational Review* 62(2), Summer 1992, 191–208.

Banks, J. A., "Multicultural Education: Development, Dimensions, and Challenges." *Phi Delta Kappan* 22, September 1993, 20.

Bergen, Doris, ed., *Play as a Medium for Learning and Development.* Portsmouth, N.H.: Heinemann, 1988.

Bernhard, Judith, Lefebvre, Marie Louise, Chud, Gyda, and Lange, Rika, *Paths to Equity: Cultural, Linguistic, and Racial Diversity in Canadian Early Childhood Education.* Toronto: York Lanes Press, 1995.

Billman, Janet, "The Native American Curriculum: Attempting Alternatives to Teepees and Headbands." *Young Children*, September 1992.

Block, Marianne N., Tabachnick, B. Robert, and Espinosa-Dulanto, Miryam, "Teacher Perspectives on the Strengths and Achievements of Young Children: Relationship to Ethnicity, Language, Gender, and Class," in Mallory, Bruce L., and New, Rebecca S., eds., *Diversity and Developmentally Appropriate Practices: Challenges for Early Childhood Education.* New York: Teachers College Press, 1994, 223–249.

Bowlby, J., *Attachment and Loss: Vol. 1: Attachment.* New York: Basic Books, 1969.

Bowman, Barbara T., and Stott, Frances M., "Understanding Development in a Cultural Context: The Challenge for Teachers," in Mallory, Bruce L., and New, Rebecca S., eds., *Diversity and Developmentally Appropriate Practices: Challenges for Early Childhood Education*. New York: Teachers College Press, 1994, 119–133.

Brazelton, T. B., "A Child Oriented Approach to Toilet Training." *Pediatrics* 29(1), January 1962.

Bredekamp, Sue, ed., *Developmental Appropriate Practice in Early Childhood Programs Serving Children From Birth Through Age 8*. Washington, D.C.: National Association for the Education of Young Children, 1987.

Brown, Joseph E., *The Spiritual Legacy of the American Indian*. New York: Crossroad Publishing, 1982.

Cajete, Gregory, *Look to the Mountain: An Ecology of Indigenous Education*. Durango, Colo.: Kivaki Press, 1994.

Campbell, Kate, "Energy Program Helps Refugees Make Transition to Life in the U.S." *PG &E Progress*, April 1985.

Carroll, Raymonde, *Cultural Misunderstandings: The French-American Experience*. Chicago: University of Chicago Press, 1988.

Caudill, W., and Winstein, H., "Maternal Care and Infant Behavior in Japan and America." *Psychiatry* 1969, 32, 12–43.

Chan, I. *The Hmong in America: Their Cultural Continuities and Discontinuities*. St. Paul, Minn.: University of Minnesota, ERIC, ED 217 105, 1981.

Chang, Hedy, *Affirming Children's Roots: Cultural and Linguistic Diversity in Early Care and Education*. San Francisco: California Tomorrow, 1993.

Chud, G., and Fahlman, R., *Early Childhood Education for a Multicultural Society: A Handbook for Educators*. Vancouver: Pacific Educational Press, 1990.

Comer, J., "Research and the Black Backlash." *American Journal of Orthopsychiatry* 40, 1970, 8–11.

Comer, J. P., and Poussaint, A. F., *Black Child Care*. New York: Simon and Schuster, 1975.

Crawford, James, *Bilingual Education: History, Politics, Theory and Practice*. Trenton, N.J.: Crane Publishing, 1989.

Delpit, Lisa, "The Silenced Dialogue: Power and Pedagogy in Educating Other People's Children." *Harvard Educational Review* 58(3), 1988, 280–298.

Derman-Sparks, Louise, "The Process of Culturally Sensitive Care," in Mangione, Peter, ed., *Infant/Toddler Caregiving: A Guide to Culturally Sensitive Care*. Sacramento, Calif.: Far West Laboratory and California Department of Education, 1995.

Derman-Sparks, Louise, and the ABC Task Force, *Antibias Curriculum: Tools for Empowering Young Children*. Washington, D.C.: National Association for the Education of Young Children, 1989.

Dorris, Michael, *Paper Trail*. New York: HarperCollins, 1994.

Dreikurs, Rudolf, and Grey, Loren, *Logical Consequences: A New Approach to Discipline*. New York: Dutton, 1990.

Dung, Trinh Ngoc, "Understanding Asian Families: A Vietnamese Perspective." *Children Today*, March-April 1984.

Duong, Thanh Binh, *A Handbook for Teachers of Vietnamese Students: Hints for Dealing with Cultural Differences in Schools*. Arlington, Va.: Center for Applied Linguisitics, 1975.

Edwards, Carolyn P., and Gandini, Lella, "Teachers' Expectations About the Timing of Developmental Skills: A Cross-Cultural Study." *Young Children*, May 1989, 15–19.

Edwards, Patricia, Fear, Kathleen L.,and Gallego, Margaret A., "Role of Parents in Responding to Issues of Linguistic and Cultural Diversity," in Garcia, Eugene E., and McLaughlin, Barry, eds., with Spokek, Bernard, and Saracho, Olivia N., *Meeting the Challenge of Linguistic and Cultural Diversity in Early Childhood Education*. New York: Teachers College Press, 1995, 141–153.

Ehling, Marta Borbon, "The Mexican American (El Chicano)," in Clark, A. L., ed., *Culture and Childrearing*. Philadelphia: F. A. Davis Company, 1981.

Fantini, M. D.,and Cardenas, R., eds., *Parenting in a Multicultural Society*. New York: Longman, 1980.

Fenichel, Emily S., and Eggbeer, Linda, *Preparing Practitioners to Work with Infants, Toddlers, and Their Families: Issues and Recommendations for the Professions*. Arlington, Va.: National Center for Clinical Infant Programs, 1990.

Fisher, Roger, and Ury, William, *Getting to Yes: Negotiating Agreement Without Giving In*. New York: Penguin Books, 1991.

France, P., "Working with Young Bilingual Children." *Early Child Development and Care* 10, 1980, 283–292.

Galinsky, Ellen, "From Our President: Why are Some Parent/Teacher Partnerships Clouded with Difficulties?" *Young Children* 45(5), July 1990, 2–3, 38–39.

Garcia, Eugene, *Understanding and Meeting the Challenge of Student Cultural Diversity*. Boston: Houghton Mifflin, 1994.

Garcia, Eugene E., and McLaughlin, Barry, eds., with Spokek, Bernard, and Saracho, Olivia N., *Meeting the Challenge of Linguistic and Cultural Diversity in Early Childhood Education*. New York: Teachers College Press, 1995.

Gardner, Howard, *Frames of Mind*. New York: Basic Books, 1983.

Gardner, Howard, *To Open Minds, Chinese Clues to the Dilemma of Contemporary Education*. New York: Basic Books, 1989.

Garrett, W. E., "The Hmong of Laos: No Place to Run." *National Geographic* 141, January 1974, 78–111.

Garrett, W. E., "Thailand: Refuge from Terror." *National Geographic* 157, May 1980, 633–642.

Genishi, Celia, and Brainard, Margaret Borrego, "Assessment of Bilingual Children: A Dilemma Seeking Solutions" in Garcia, Eugene E., and McLaughlin, Barry, eds., with Spokek, Bernard, and Saracho, Olivia N., *Meeting the Challenge of Linguistic and Cultural Diversity in Early Childhood Education*. New York: Teachers College Press, 1995, 49–62.

Gerber, M., ed., *Manual for Resources for Infant Educarers*. Los Angeles: Resources for Infant Educarers, 1988.

Gomez, Mary Louise, "Breaking Silences: Building New Stories of Classroom Life Through Teacher Transformation," in Kessler, Shirley A., and Swadener, Beth Blue, eds., *Reconceptualizing the Early Childhood Curriculum: Beginning the Dialogue*. New York: Teachers College Press, 1992, 165–188.

Gonzalez-Mena, Janet, "English as a Second Language for Preschool Children," in Cazden, C. B., ed., *Lanquage in Early Childhood Education*, rev. ed., Washington, D.C.: NAEYC, 1981, 127–132.

Gonzalez-Mena, Janet. *A Caregiver's Guide to Routines in Infant-Toddler Care*. Sacramento, Calif.: State of California, Department of Education, Child Development Division, The Center for Child and Family Studies, Far West Laboratory for Educational Research and Development, 1990.

Gonzalez-Mena, Janet, "Do You Have Cultural Tunnel Vision?" *Child Care Information Exchange*, July-August 1991, 29–31.

Gonzalez-Mena, Janet, "Taking a Culturally Sensitive Approach in Infant-Toddler Programs." *Young Children* 47(2), January 1992, 4–9.

Gonzalez-Mena, Janet, *The Child in the Family and the Community*. New York: Merrill, 1993.

Gonzalez-Mena, Janet, "The Man Who Ordered a Tortilla and Got an Omelette," in *Family Information Services*, Minneapolis, Minn.: Family Information Services, 1995, pp. M & O, 5–6.

Gonzalez-Mena, Janet, "Cultural Sensitivity in Routine CaregivingTasks," in Mangione, Peter, ed., *Infant/Toddler Caregiving: A Guide to Culturally Sensitive Care*. Sacramento, Calif.: Far West Laboratory and California Department of Education, 1995.

Gonzalez-Mena, Janet, and Eyer, D., *Infants, Toddlers, and Caregivers*. Mountain View, Calif.: Mayfield Publishing Company, 1989.

Gonzalez-Mena, Janet, and Stonehouse, Anne, "In the Child's Best Interests." *Child Care Information Exchange*, November 1995, 17–20.

Greenberg, Polly, "Teaching About Native Americans or Teaching About People, Including Native Americans?" *Young Children*, September 1992.

Greenman, Jim, "Living in the Real World: Diversity and Conflict." *Exchange*, October 1989, 11.

Gudykunst, W. BV., ed., *Intercultural Communication Theory: Current Perspectives*. Beverly Hills, Calif.: Sage, 1983.

Hakuta, K., *Mirror of Language*. New York: Basic Books, 1986.

Hale, Janice E., "An African-American Early Childhood Education Program: Visions for Children," in Kessler, Shirley A., and Swadener, Beth Blue, eds., *Reconceptualizing the Early Childhood Curriculum: Beginning the Dialogue*. New York: Teachers College Press, 1992, 205–224.

Hale, Janice E., *Black Children: Their Roots, Culture and Learning Styles*. Baltimore, Md.: The Johns Hopkins University Press, 1986.

Hale, Janice E., "The Transmission of Cultural Values to Young African American Children." *Young Children* 46(6), September 1991, 7–15.

Hall, Edward T., *Beyond Culture*. Garden City, N.Y.: Anchor Books, 1977.

Heath, Shirley Brice, *Ways with Words: Language, Life and Work in Communities and Classrooms*. Cambridge, Mass.: Cambridge University Press, 1983.

Hildebrand, Verna, Phenice, Lillan A., Gray, Mary M., and Hines, Rebecca P., *Knowing and Serving Diverse Families*. Englewood Cliffs, N.J.: Prentice-Hall, 1996.

Holtzman, Wayne H., Diaz-Guerrero, Rogelio, and Swartz, Jon D., *Personality Development in Two Cultures: A Cross-Cultural Longitudinal Study of School Children in Mexico and the United States.* Austin, Tex.: University of Texas Press, 1975, 359.

Hopson, Darlene Powell, and Hopson, Derek S., *Different and Wonderful: Raising Black Children in a Race-Conscious Society.* New York: Prentice-Hall, 1990.

Howard, G. R., "Whites in Multicultural Education: Rethinking Our Role." *Phi Delta Kappan*, September 1993, 36–41.

Hsu, Francis L. K., *Americans and Chinese: Purpose and Fulfillment in Great Civilizations.* Garden City, N.Y.: The Natural History Press, 1970.

Jipson, J., "Extending the Discourse on Developmental Appropriateness: A Developmental Perspective." *Early Education and Development* 2(2), 1991, 95–108.

Jones, Elizabeth, *Teaching Adults: An Active Learning Approach.* Washington, D.C.: National Association for the Education of Young Children, 1987.

Jones, Elizabeth, and Derman Sparks, Louise, "Meeting the Challenge of Diversity." *Young Children* 47(2), January 1992, 12–18.

Jones, Elizabeth,and Nimmo, John, *Emergent Curriculum.* Washington, D.C.: National Association for Education of Young Children, 1994.

Kagan, Jerome, *The Nature of the Child.* New York: Basic Books, 1984.

Kawagley, A. Oscar, *A Yupiaz Worldview: A Pathway to Ecology and Spirit.* Prospect Heights, Ill.: Waveland Press, 1995.

Kendall, F., *Diversity in the Classroom.* New York: Teachers College Press, 1983.

Kennedy, Geraldine, ed., *From the Center of the Earth: Stories out of the Peace Corps.* Santa Monica, Calif.: Clover Park Press, 1991.

Kessler, S.,and Swaderner, B., *Reconceptualizing the Early Childhood Curriculum, Beginning the Dialogue.* New York: Teachers College Press, 1992.

Kitano, Margie K., "Early Childhood Education for Asian American Children." *Young Children*, January 1980, 13–26.

Knight, George P., Bernal, Martha E., and Carlo, Gustavo, "Socialization and the Development of Cooperative, Competitive, and Individualistic Behaviors Among Mexican American Children," in Garcia, Eugene E., and McLaughlin, Barry, eds., with Spokek, Bernard, and Saracho, Olivia N., *Meeting the Challenge of Linguistic and Cultural Diversity in Early Childhood Education.* New York: Teachers College Press, 1995, 85–102.

Ladson-Billings, Gloria, *The Dreamkeepers: Successful Teachers of African American Children.* San Francisco: Jossey-Bass, 1994.

Leach, P., *Your Baby and Child From Birth to Age Five.* New York: Alfred A. Knopf, 1987.

Lee, Dorothy, *Freedom and Culture.* A Spectrum Book, Englewood Cliffs, N.J.: Prentice-Hall, 1959.

Lee, Fong Yun, "Asian Parents as Partners." *Young Children*, March 1995, 4–8.

Lee, Joann, *Asian Americans.* New York: New Press, 1992.

Lefley, H., and Pedersen, P., eds., *Cross-Cultural Training for Mental Health Professionals.* Springfield, Ill.: Charles C. Thomas, 1986.

Levine, Robert A., "Child Rearing as Cultural Adaptation," in Leiderman, P. Herbert, Tulkin, Steven, R., and Rosenfeld, Anne, eds., *Culture and Infancy: Variations in the Human Experience.* New York and San Francisco: Academic Press, 1977.

Levine, Robert A., "A Cross-cultural Perspective on Parenting," in Fantini, M.D., and Cardenas, R., eds., *Parenting in a Multicultural Society.* New York: Longman, 1980, 17–26.

Lieberman, Alicia F., "Concerns of Immigrant Families," in Mangione, Peter, ed., *Infant/Toddler Caregiving: A Guide to Culturally Sensitive Care.* Sacramento, Calif.: Far West Laboratory and California Department of Education, 1995.

Liederman, P. H., et al. *Culture and Infancy: Variations in Human Experience.* New York: Academic Press, 1977.

Little Soldier, Lee, "Working with Native American Children." *Young Children* 47(6), September 1992, 15–17.

Lubeck, Sally, *The Sandbox Society: Early Education in Black and White America.* Philadelphia: The Falmer Press, 1985.

Lynch, Eleanor W., and Hanson, Marci J., *Developing Cross-Cultural Competence: A Guide for Working with Young Children and Their Families.* Baltimore, Md.: Paul H. Brookes Publishing, 1992.

Makin, Laurie, Campbell, Julie, and Diaz, Criss Jones, *One Childhood, Many Languages.* Pymble, NSW, Australia: HarperEducational, 1995.

Mallory, Bruce L.,and New, Rebecca S., eds., *Diversity and Developmentally Appropriate Practices: Challenges for Early Childhood Education.* New York: Teachers College Press, 1994.

Mander, Jerry, *In the Absence of the Sacred.* San Francisco: Sierra Club Books, 1991.

Mangione, Peter, ed., *Infant/Toddler Caregiving: A Guide to Culturally Sensitive Care.* Sacramento, Calif.: Far West Laboratory and California Department of Education, 1995.

Matthiessen, Neba, *The Hmong: A Multicultural Study.* Fairfield, Calif.: Fairfield-Suisun Unified School District, 1987.

McCracken, Janet Brown, *Valuing Diversity: The Primary Years.* Washington, D.C.: National Association for the Education of Young Children, 1993.

McIntosh, Peggy, *White Privilege and Male Privilege: A Personal Account of Coming to See Correspondences Through Work in Women's Studies.* Working Paper No. 189. Wellesley, Mass.: Wellesley College Center for Research on Women, 1988.

Means, Russell, *Where White Men Fear to Tread.* New York: St. Martin's Press, 1995.

Medicine, Beatrice, "Child Socialization Among Native Americans: The Lakota (Sioux) in Cultural Context." *Wicazo Sa Review* 1(2), Fall 1985, 23–28.

Miner, Barbara, "Teachers, Culture, and Power: An Interview with African-American Educator Lisa Delpit." *Rethinking Schools*, March/April 1992, 14-16.

Mistry, Jayanthi, "Culture and Learning in Infancy," in Mangione, Peter, ed., *Infant/Toddler Caregiving: A Guide to Culturally Sensitive Care.* Sacramento, Calif.: Far West Laboratory and California Department of Education, 1995.

Morelli, G., Rogoff, B., and Oppenheim, D., "Cultural Variation in Infants' Sleeping Arrangements: Questions of Independence." *Developmental Psychology* 28(4), July 1992, 604–619.

Morrow, Robert D., "Cultural Differences—Be Aware!" *Academic Therapy* 23, November 1987, 2.

Morrow, Robert D., "What's in a Name? In Particular, a Southeast Asian Name?" *Young Children*, September 1989, 20–23.

Native American Parent Preschool Curriculum Guide. Oakland, Calif.: Office of Native American Programs, Division of Educational Development and Services, 1986.

Neihardt, John G., *Black Elk Speaks.* New York: Pocket Books, 1972.

Neugebauer, Bonnie, ed., *Alike and Different: Exploring our Humanity with Young Children.* Washington, D.C.: National Association for the Education of Young Children, 1992.

Nourot, Patricia, Monighan, Scales, Barbara, Van Horn, Judith, and Almy, Milly, *Looking at Children's Play: A Bridge Between Theory and Practice.* New York: Teachers College Press, 1987.

Nugent, J. Kevin, "Cross-Cultural Studies of Child Development: Implications for Clinicians." *Zero to Three* 15(2), October/November 1994, 1–7.

Ogbu, John U., "Understanding Cultural Diversity and Learning," *Educational Researcher,* November 1992, 5–14.

Outsama, Kao, *Laotian Themes.* Philadelphia: Temple University, 1977.

Phillips, Carol Brunson, "Nurturing Diversity for Today's Children and Tomorrow's Leaders." *Young Children* 43(2), 1988, 42–47.

Phillips, Carol Brunson, "The Movement of African-American Children Through Sociocultural Contexts: A Case of Conflict Resolution," in Malloy, Bruce L., and New, Rebecca S., eds., *Diversity and Developmentally Appropriate Practices: Challenges for Early Childhood Education.* New York: Teachers College Press, 1994, 137–154.

Phillips, Carol Brunson, "Culture: A Process that Empowers," in Mangione, Peter, ed., *Infant/Toddler Caregiving: A Guide to Culturally Sensitive Care.* Sacramento, Calif.: Far West Laboratory and California Department of Education, 1995.

Phillips, Carol Brunson, and Cooper, Renatta M., "Cultural Dimensions of Feeding Relationships." *Zero to Three,* June 1992, 10–13.

Procidano, Mary E., and Fisher, Celia B., *Contemporary Families: A Handbook for School Professionals.* New York: Teachers College Press, 1992.

Rael, Joseph, *Being and Vibration,* Tulsa, Okla.: Council Oak Books, 1993.

Ramirez, M., and Castenada, A., *Cultural Democracy, Bicognitive Development and Education.* New York: Academic Press, 1974.

Ramsey, Patricia, and Derman-Sparks, Louise, "Viewpoint: Multicultural Education Reaffirmed." *Young Children* 39(2), January 1992, 10–11.

Rashid, H. B., "Promoting Biculturalism in Young African-American Children." *Young Children* 39(2), 1984, 12–23.

Rodriguez, R., *The Hunger of Memory: The Education of Richard Rodriguez.* New York: Bantam Books, 1983.

Root, Maria, Ho, Christine, and Sue, Stanley, "Issues in the Training of Counselors for Asian Americans," in Lefley, H., and Pedersen, P, eds., *Cross-Cultural Training for Mental Health Professionals.* Springfield, Ill.: Charles C. Thomas, 1986.

Ross, Allen C. (Ehanamani), *Mitakuye Oyasin: We Are All Related.* Denver, Colo.: Wichoni Waste, 1989.

Sandoval, M., and De La Roza, M., "A Cultural Perspective for Serving the Hispanic Client," in Lefley, Harriet, and Pedersen, Paul, *Cross-Cultural Training for Mental Health Professionals.* Springfield, Ill.: Charles C. Thomas, 1986.

Sandoz, M., *Crazy Horse: The Stange Man of the Oglalas.* Lincoln, Nebr.: University of Nebraska Press, 1961.

Saracho, Olivia N., and Spodek, Bernard, "Preparing Teachers for Early Childhood Programs," in Garcia, Eugene E., and McLaughlin, Barry, eds., with Spokek, Bernard, and Saracho, Olivia N., *Meeting the Challenge of Linguistic and Cultural Diversity in Early Childhood Education.* New York: Teachers College Press, 1995, 154–166.

Saracho, O. N., and Spodek, B., eds., *Understanding the Multicultural Experience in Early Childhood Education.* Washington, D.C.: National Association for the Education of Young Children, 1983.

Sholtys, Katherine Cullen, "A New Language, A New Life: Recommendations for Teachers of Non-English-Speaking Children Newly Entering the Program." *Young Children,* March 1989, 76–77.

Slapin, Beverly, and Seale, Doris, *Books without Bias: Through Indian Eyes.* Berkeley, Calif.: Oyate, 1988.

Snowden, Lonnie R., "Toward Evaluation of Black Psycho-Social Competence," in Sue, Stanley, and Moore, Thom, eds., *The Pluralistic Society.* New York: Human Sciences Press, 1984.

Sodetaini-Shibata, "The Japanese American," in Clark, A. L, ed., *Culture and Childrearing.* Philadelphia: F. A. Davis Company, 1981.

Soto, Lourdes Diaz, "Understanding Bicultural/Bilingual Young Children." *Young Children,* January 1991.

Soto, Lourdes Diaz, and Smrekar, Jocelynn L., "The Politics of Early Bilingual Education," in Kessler, Shirley A., and Swadener, Beth Blue, eds., *Reconceptualizing the Early Childhood Curriculum: Beginning the Dialogue.* New York: Teachers College Press, 1992, 189–202.

Spencer, Margaret Beale, Brookins, Geraldine Kearse, and Recharde, Allen Walter, eds., *Beginnings: The Social and Affective Development of Black Children.* Hillsdale, N.J.: Erlbaum, 1985.

Stern, Daniel N., *The Interpersonal World of the Infant.* New York: Basic Books, 1985.

Stewart, Edward C., *American Cultural Patterns: A Cross-Cultural Perspective.* Yarmouth, Maine: Intercultural Press, 1972.

Storti, Craig, *The Art of Crossing Cultures.* Yarmouth, Maine: Intercultural Press, 1990.

Stringfellow, L., Liem, N. D., and Liem, L., in Clark, Ann L. ed., *Culture and Childrearing.* Philadelphia: F. A. Davis Company, 1981.

Sturm, Connie, "Intercultural Communication in Child Care: Creating Parent-Teacher Dialogue." Master's Thesis, 1995.

Sue, Stanley, and Moore, Thom, eds., *The Pluralistic Society*. New York: Human Sciences Press, 1984.

Sung, B. L. *Chinese Immigrant Children in New York City: The Experience of Adjustment*. New York: Center for Migration Studies, 1987.

Tedla, Elleni, *Sankofa: African Thought and Education*. New York: Peter Lang, 1995.

Thorman, E. B., and Browder S., *Born Dancing*. New York: Harper & Row, 1987.

Tizard, Barbara, and Hughes, Martin, *Young Children Learning*. Cambridge, Mass.: Harvard University Press, 1984.

Tobin, Joseph J., Wu, David Y. H., and Davidson, Dana H., *Preschool in Three Cultures*. New Haven, Conn.: Yale University Press, 1989.

Tronick, E. Z., Morelli, G. A., and Winn S., "Multiple Caretaking of Efe (Pygmy) Infants." *American Anthropologist* 89, 1987, 96–106.

Trueba, H. T., *Raising Silent Voices*. Boston: Heinle and Heinle, 1989.

Villarruel, Francisco A., Imig, David R., and Kostelnik, Marjorie J., "Diverse Families," in Garcia, Eugene G., and McLaughlin, Barry, eds., with Spokek, Bernard, and Saracho, Olivia N., *Meeting the Challenge of Linguistic and Cultural Diversity in Early Childhood Education*. New York: Teachers College Press, 1995, 103–124.

Wagner, Daniel A., and Stevenson, Harold W., eds., *Cultural Perspectives on Child Development*. San Francisco: W. H. Freeman and Company, 1982.

Wardel, Francis, "Are You Sensitive to Interracial Children's Special Identity Needs?" *Young Children*, January 1987, 53–59.

Wardel, Francis, "Endorsing Children's Differences: Meeting the Needs of Adopted Minority Children." *Young Children*, July 1990, 44–46.

Werner, E. *Cross-Cultural Child Development: A View from the Planet Earth*. Monterey, Calif.: Brooks/Cole Publishing Company, 1979.

Williams, Leslie R., "Developmentally Appropriate Practice and Cultural Values: A Case in Point," in Mallory, Bruce L., and New, Rebecca S., eds., *Diversity and Developmentally Appropriate Practices: Challenges for Early Childhood Education*. New York: Teachers College Press, 1994, 155–165.

Wong-Fillmore, Lilly, "When Learning a Second Language Means Losing the First." *Early Childhood Research Quarterly* 6, 1991.

Yntema, Sharon, *Vegetarian Children*. Ithaca, N.Y.: McBooks Press, 1987.

York, Stacy, *Roots and Wings: Affirming Culture in Early Childhood Programs*. St. Paul, Minn.: Redleaf Press, 1991.

Young, V. H., "Family and Childhood in a Southern Negro Community." *American Anthropologist* 72, 1970, 269–288.

Young, V. H., "A Black American Socialization Pattern." *American Ethnologist*, 1, 1974, 405–413.

Index